GROWING UP PROUD

GROWING UP PROUD

A Parent's Guide To The Psychological Care Of Children With Disabilities

JAMES E. LINDEMANN, PH.D.
SALLY J. LINDEMANN, M.S.

WARNER BOOKS

A Warner Communications Company

Grateful acknowledgment is given to The Crippled Children's Division for permission to use the instrument *Portland Tracking System for Adult Living* © 1981 in this book.

Warner Books, Inc., 666 Fifth Avenue, New York, NY 10103

Ⓦ A Warner Communications Company

Printed in the United States of America
First Printing: July 1988
10 9 8 7 6 5 4 3 2 1

Interior Design By: Judy Allan (The Designing Woman Concepts)

Library of Congress Cataloging-in-Publication Data
Lindemann, James E. (James Earl), 1927–
   Growing up proud: a parent's guide to the psychological care of children with disabilities / James E. Lindemann, Ph.D. and Sally J. Lindemann. M. S.
      p. cm.
   Includes index.
   ISBN 0-446-38682-0
   1. Parents of handicapped children—United States.
   2. Handicapped children—United States—Psychology. 3. Parenting—United States. 4. Handicapped children—Care—United States.
   I. Lindemann, Sally J.   II. Title.
   [DNLM: 1. Handicapped—psychology—popular works.
   2. Rehabilitation—in infancy & childhood—popular works.   WS
   105.5.H2 L743g]
   HQ759.913.L56 1988
   649'.15—dc19
   DNLM/DLC
   for Library of Congress   87-28058
                                                              CIP

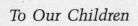

To Our Children

Contents

We are thankful to the following professionals, parents and persons with disabilities who were kind enough to read the manuscript of this book and to enrich it with their comments: Sylvia Betts, Barbara Boas, Larry Brown, Virginia Danzer, Ann Garner, Ingrid Leckliter, David MacFarlane, Maren Peterson, Marilyn Rich, Cheryl Saunders, Robin Stephens, Leif Terdal, and Sue Wright.

We are deeply grateful to our colleagues and fellow staff members at the Crippled Children's Division of the Oregon Health Sciences University and at the District and Regional Assessment Center of the Portland School District. The insights and experiences they have shared with us have provided much of the substance of our professional growth and perspective. We owe special thanks to the Department of Psychological Medicine, University of Glasgow, Scotland, where a major part of this book was written.

Our greatest debt is to the children and families with whom we have worked over the years and to our own three children and our grandchildren. They have taught us the wisdom of their selfhood.

James and Sally Lindemann

Introduction

This book is intended to provide parents with information that will help them to deal with their own feelings about disability and to develop attitudes and expectations that will allow their children to use their abilities to the maximum, to feel good about themselves, and to grow up proud. It has practical suggestions about day-to-day living, from how to inform the relatives about the birth of a child with a disability, to techniques of child training, to the particular needs of the disabled teenager. Most of the principles apply to all children, with or without disability, although special attention is paid to some matters that parents of disabled children often find difficult. The book is intended to provide guidelines and principles rather than be a comprehensive manual. It is short and written in a style that is straightforward and easy to read. It includes references to sources of further information on many topics and suggestions as to when it is appropriate to get professional advice.

The book is divided into two main sections. Part I begins with the arrival of the disabled child or the beginning of the disability. It discusses accepting the child, dealing with professionals, obtaining understandable information, and introducing the child to home, family (including brothers and sisters), and friends. It goes through the life stages of toddler, schoolchild, teenager, and young adult, discussing the problems and joys that emerge and making suggestions about appropriate activities as well as services that might be helpful. The information in Part I is intended to apply to children of all ages (Chapter Two, for example, on the new child, contains suggestions about the newly diagnosed child of any age). We suggest that you read the entire section. It contains useful principles throughout.

Part II consists of thirteen chapters on a variety of topics including child training, school, severe disability, and the effects of sensory impairment. It contains a chapter especially addressed to the personal needs of all parents, as well as one for the single parent. We recommend familiarizing yourself with these chapters and then using them for reference as needed.

We believe that the guidelines in the book will apply, in principle, to all children with disability. We recognize that children's capacities will vary according to the type and severity of their disabling condition. For example, care may be needed in setting limits and expectations for those with cognitive impairment (such as mental retardation or brain damage) that might reduce the children's level of comprehension, judgment, or capacity for self-responsibility. Children with impaired hearing or vision may have specific limitations in some situations. We feel strongly, however, that the principle of maximizing independence and self-reliance applies to all and that it is important to adapt the level of expectation to the individual child, if necessary, but not to write off any area of activity as impossible for any children, regardless of the severity of their impairment.

This book applies equally to both sexes. We have sought to be evenhanded in writing it, but also found that we could not make it individualized and personal enough without using pronouns like *she* and *he.* Our solution has been to vary their use throughout the book. We believe we have accomplished this fairly and hope you will be comfortable with the result.

There are anecdotes and examples throughout the nineteen chapters. They are based on experiences we have had or people we have known. In some instances a story may combine incidents that happened to several people. The names and other identifying characteristics have been changed to protect the privacy of individuals. The events, however, are true.

Our intention has been to make this book practical and readable as well as consistent with current professional principles. It is based on the professional experience each of us has had with a large number of disabled children and their parents, our awareness of the accumulated knowledge in the fields of psychology and physical disability, and our personal experience in rearing our own three children. We owe a great debt to each of those sources. We invite you to add to the usefulness of our practice, and of further editions of this book, by sharing with us your experiences, comments, and suggestions.

James E. Lindemann
Sally J. Lindemann
Portland, Oregon
October 1987

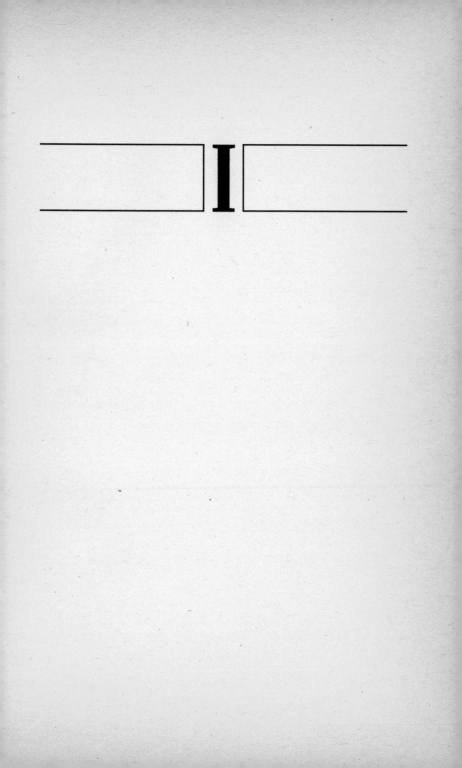

I

1

Life Is a Parade

Some days are very special, such as the day a child is born. No other day will be the same to the child. No other child will be the same, either. No one else will have the same combination of blue or brown eyes, straight or curly hair, Daddy's nose or Mother's smile. If children could focus their eyes on Day One, they might be just as eager as anyone else to see what they look like in the mirror. They've been trying their best to grow up for months. They'll continue to try their best. Given the opportunity they'll grow, expand their world, and develop ever more skills. Mom and Dad's job is to provide what is needed in the way of nurture and space, and to enjoy watching it happen. No one else will do it in quite the same way. No one can really predict the outcome with any certainty, nor should they. What a day—the first day of the parade through life!

No one wants rain on that parade. Everyone's aim is set on perfect. Perfect? Does that mean *really* perfect? Like me? Like you? Well—er, maybe like those perfect guys on TV. What is less than perfect? Being short? Fat? Tone deaf? Wearing glasses? Uncoordinated? Stubborn? Homely? Walking with a limp? Unable to read? Not walking at all? There are degrees of "imperfection." We have them, our family has them, our friends have them.

People all around us have "imperfections" and "disabilities" that we take for granted, all the time thinking of their owners as just plain folks we love, admire, and respect. Somehow, with them, we have avoided the labels IMPERFECT and DISABLED.

This book is about children who could be seen as wearing BIG labels. It is written for the parents, relatives, and friends of persons who are called disabled. They have conditions with names such as cerebral palsy, spina bifida, paraplegia, quadriplegia, congenital heart disease, mental retardation, muscular dystrophy, hemophilia, blindness, deafness, and so on. The book will describe families who have had such members; how they felt; what they did that was good; what they did that was wrong or foolish; what common pitfalls they experienced; what some of the principles are that seem to work. Most of all, it will try to describe an attitude or philosophy (and steps for carrying it out) that will make life enjoyable for both parents and children. You have heard that the optimist sees the pitcher as half full, while the pessimist sees it as half empty. The same set of abilities and life accomplishments can lead some children and their families to be proud and excited and others to be disappointed and discontent. We will examine the ways through which they arrive at these different points of view.

2

IN THE BEGINNING
The New Child

When parents learn that their child has a disability, a common reaction is disbelief. Something must be wrong: the diagnosis is a mistake, or it's the wrong child. You feel stunned, unable to think clearly, perhaps barely able to move, even though your impulse may be to do something *now*. It is human to react to a sudden loss with denial or even outrage. Not knowing much about the child or the disability, you may see the situation as more devastating or impossible than it really is, which adds to the intensity of your feelings. It is something that you could not anticipate and did not choose, and therefore it is a hurt that seems undeserved and unfair. You feel badly used. These are feelings you should share and discuss with people close to you, such as your family or friends, perhaps a counselor or religious mentor. They are honest feelings that are warranted and need to be expressed but that should shortly be brought under your control, rather than having them control you.

Such an event is a time to think and act slowly and to get as much information as you can. You may not be able to remember or understand all the details the first time you hear them. Take every opportunity you can get to hear them again and to learn more. Write down the questions you want to ask. Most disabilities are complicated; they may have different causes, may have different levels of severity, and may require different kinds of treatment. The course for your child may not be clear in the beginning, and you can be sure that his or her needs will change at different stages of development. Don't hesitate to ask questions, even if you're afraid they're obvious or "dumb." The wise professional will know that it will be hard for you to "hear" and understand, will take the time to explain things clearly, and will be willing to explain more than once. Ask questions until you do understand.

You may feel impatient or angry; try not to let that interfere with getting information. Don't make important decisions while you are dazed with disbelief, hot with anger, or numb with fatigue. Learning about your child and her disability will take place over time, and most decisions don't need to be rushed. Seek the opportunity for repeated discussions with professional staff, and ask for additional appointments if necessary. In the meantime, spend time with your child; the fact that she squeaks, smiles, cries, or wriggles will let you know that she's a great deal like other kids and will be in the future. Plus, like all the rest of us, she'll have some special charms all her own. Everyone who gets to know her close up will know that she's more than a diagnosis.

We may seem to be saying that accepting your child with her disability should be an easy process; we would be less than honest if we said that. You may well feel grief, sadness about those things that your child will miss, disappointment about some of the dreams you had for this child that may not be achieved. You may feel guilt: What have I done wrong? What should I have done differently? This can be compounded if one family member chooses (often irrationally) to fix blame. You may also feel anger, something has been taken from something has been done to your child. Why you? Why your child? A feeling of resentment is almost unavoidable, complicated by the fact that the target for resentment may not be clear. God? Fate? Heredity? Yourself? Your mate? The professionals? The child? You may worry. A common cause for worry is the financial impact, the cost of care for a child with a disability. While there is usually some assistance with this, it will also represent a burden. You should not feel guilty about considering costs as you go about getting services for your child.

Disappointment, grief, worry, resentment, and anger are all honest feelings to which you are entitled and that you should share with those close to you, such as your mate, your relatives, and your friends. In some cases you may need to obtain professional help to deal with these feelings. Try not to let them interfere with acquiring the information you need and carrying out the actions that are required for your child. Try not to allow grief or anger to distort your decisions. In dealing with professionals, you may sometimes need to be assertive to get the information you need, but try not to let that assertiveness erupt into anger that can disrupt communication.

As parents first begin to learn about the disability of a child, they may ask themselves if all this information is accurate, if all these recommendations are the best ones. They may ask if we are doing right by our child? Are we getting the best? In many instances the parents know that the professionals they are dealing with are recognized, competent, and sincere. They feel satisfied with the diagnosis, treatment, and professional support they are receiving, and ready to go on from there. Sometimes genuine doubts, the drive to be absolutely certain, or difficulty in accepting the disability and its implica-

tions will lead a family to seek other opinions. That is a
legitimate right and, in some instances, an appropriate
thing to do. It should be done in a manner that does not
detract from your child's ongoing care. The first thing to
do is to tell the professionals with whom you are working that you would like to obtain a second opinion. You
may want to ask for their suggestions regarding others to
consult, or you may wish to make that choice based on
independent information and advice. In any event, you
should let them know that you are seeing someone else
and let the new professionals you consult know about
your previous contacts. Whatever professional staff you
finally choose for continued services should know that
you have seen others and be provided with copies of
their reports.

In some instances even a third opinion may be
appropriate, rarely more. Shopping around for a more
favorable diagnosis or prognosis consumes time and money and may lead you to consider programs of dubious
worth. In seeking consultation, always be certain that
the persons you see are known in the community, licensed or certified in their field, and specialized in the
disability area of your concern. They should be able to
document the value of their approach. Avoid well-
advertised but unproven methods or theories. *There are
seldom simple answers to complicated problems, and
methods which seem to be too good to be true may be
just that.* Because you could be under emotional pressure or stress at this time, it may be wise to discuss your
decision with others whose judgment you trust.

In the end, it will be important that you be reasonably satisfied with your child's diagnosis, the treatment
that is recommended, and the general expectations you
have been given (no one can tell you *precisely* what your

child may or may not achieve). It is also important that both parents (or all primary caretakers) view the child's disability in ways that are compatible, if not identical. We have been working with the family of Emma, who needs leg braces to assist her walking. Mother is working with the therapist to help Emma adjust to this change and to see that she wears them regularly. Dad is bothered by the way his little girl looks in "those funny-looking things" and disagrees (in front of Emma) about when she should be expected to wear them. The parents are currently involved in counseling because it is important to resolve this issue as well as several other differences they have about Emma and her care.

Children suffer the most when parents differ drastically in their ideas about the seriousness of the disability or the kind of treatment that is necessary. Maintaining open communication while learning about the disability, with plenty of consultation from professionals, is helpful in avoiding such differences. For that reason, it is also desirable for both parents to be present for professional consultations, or to alternate the responsibility for taking the child in for treatment or examination. If serious differences remain between parents about the way they view their child's disability, they should seek professional counseling to assist in resolving those differences. It is very important to the child's future!

After you have learned (primarily from professionals) the basic information about your child's disability (diagnosis, recommended treatment, general outlook for the future), it is time to seek the practical information, suggestions, and support that can come from other parents. Parents who have experience in living with a child whose disability is similar to your child's can be a gold

mine of ideas as well as a source of reassurance,
forewarning, and wisdom. They usually provide friendship and often will provide hands-on help if needed.
Your professional consultants (especially social workers,
psychologists, or physicians) may help you to make such
contacts. In many areas there are organized support
groups for the major types of disabilities. They are
worthwhile for the information and support provided by
regular meetings, for their newsletters, and as means of
access to parents with concerns similar to yours. Do not
let shyness or embarrassment keep you from the first
meeting—every parent started where you are.

In establishing close personal contacts it is generally better if you deal with more than one set of parents
in order to get more than one point of view. They should
be parents who appear to be reasonably successful in
meeting their problems and who are constructive in
their approach to dealing with their children, to assisting
others, and to the pursuit of advocacy in the community.
Be cautious with people who are angry, who want to
take over the whole problem for you, or who appear to
have their own axe to grind.

Early in this process of learning about and caring for
your special child you will find yourself wondering how
to present that child to your friends, relatives, and the
public. What to say to Grandma, Grandpa, and the others
who have been awaiting the birth? The worst thing to do
is to say that the child is perfect—no problem. The next
worst thing to say is nothing—leaving them to fill in
with all kinds of thoughts and fears. If some of these
folks (grandparents, for example) are going to be involved
closely and frequently in the child's life, it would be
good to include them in some of the dealings with your

professional staff. That way they can learn the basic information for themselves, ask questions, and hear the positive side of things as well as the negatives that they might imagine. In this time of difficulty for you, you may be experiencing a range of feelings; however, the more matter-of-fact but factual you can be in giving out information, the better. This is not to deny your concern and care but to include the message that this will be a child who is different in some ways and not so different in many others. The most serious emotional problems in later life appear to occur in children whose families attempt to deny that there is *any* disability or exaggerate its effect and rear the child as an overprotected invalid, unexposed to the hazards and joys of living. Where the disability is denied, the child may feel pressure to compete where she cannot fairly be expected to do so and that it is her fault if she fails. She may also conclude that disability is something shameful, something to be hidden. Where the disability is exaggerated, she may devalue herself and never attempt to develop her full capacities. Regardless of disability, the child will grow up, laugh, get in trouble, make accomplishments, have failures, be a burden, and be a joy—like most children. The sooner your friends and relatives get to know the child through real and frequent contacts, the better. Such contacts will mean much more than diagnoses or predictions.

There is one group that is most special in this matter of accepting a special child: the child's brothers and sisters. Hopefully they have been following Mama's pregnancy and awaiting the birth. They need to be told about their new brother or sister as fully as possible, with explanations they can understand. They will need plenty of opportunity to ask questions. They should be given a simple functional description of the baby's difficulties, that she will need some special help but that things are going to turn out all right.

The needs of the brothers and sisters should not be forgotten during this busy period. Mom and Dad should attempt to find small pieces of time just for them (as individuals and in a group if there is more than one). Care needs to be taken, of course, to see to their ongoing needs such as meals, clean clothing, school and schoolwork, and in the case of teenagers, attendance at important events. Life will go on; even though their little brother or sister is special, no one should have to miss the Junior Prom.

Having a brother or sister with a disability can be enriching to children, a living experience in the value of people who are "different." They can learn that little Bill needs help in getting up steps but sure can be fun in a card game and can catch fish better than anyone else in the family. Brothers and sisters can help and can provide a youngster's point of view as well as be a friend and companion. They should be helped to do so without giving up activities or a circle of friends of their own.

This last point is an important one for all members of the family: to maintain some identity and activities of your own. If this is done, despite the obstacles (which may be real), the final results will be enrichment of the life of all as the child is brought home and into the family.

3

THE CHILD AT HOME
The Infant and Toddler Years

Taking a new child home is a marvelous and challenging experience filled with pleasure, awe, and anxiety—the more so if it is your first child. Every new parent wonders, What happens now? What will the baby need? How do I tell? Can I do it? Who do I turn to? Although (as young mothers will tell you), you wind up doing most of it yourself, it is nice to have someone to turn to for comfort and advice. Such help is usually not too hard to find. If Grandmother or Aunt Jane is not available, an experienced friend or neighbor frequently is. Professionals such as the pediatrician or the visiting nurse may be consulted when the problem is a particularly difficult one. Some hospital nurseries will answer over-the-phone questions regarding minor problems. They may be able to reassure the parent that what seemed to be a big problem can be solved easily or that something unusual is occurring and the pediatrician should be consulted.

In addition to the help itself, there is a particular

psychological advantage to having assistance from someone else in caring for your infant. Each time you hand the child to another person to be cuddled, fed, or comforted, you are expanding his social horizons and making him more flexible. This is an important first step in the climb to independence. It is continued a month or two later when you first leave him with a mature, trusted babysitter, and on through other life experiences that teach him to get along with others.

Mary Hennings's daughter Jenny was born with spina bifida. Mr. Henning was a truck driver who was away from home for long periods of time. Jenny was a sweet baby and Mary loved caring for her. She needed a lot of care, especially because of several surgeries. The care was special, and Mary knew that others wouldn't do things just the way Jenny liked them, so she did them herself. Sometimes Mary's sister Helen would help, and Jenny liked her, so that was okay. Then Helen moved away to go to college. Jenny would cry even when the visiting nurse tried to feed her. After a while Mary found herself trapped. She could not leave Jenny at all, and Jenny seemed to be getting more finicky about things every day. In a situation where only one person (usually the mother) provides care, the baby will very soon accept care only from that person. This can create in the child dependence and inflexibility that can become a greater impairment than the physical disability itself.

Mary's problem was solved with some consultation and a good bit of help from others. Her husband arranged his schedule so he could be home for a week, and during that time he provided care for Jenny at least once or twice each day. Helen came home on vacation and provided some help several days. Mary gave Jenny some of her usual care so she would know Mother had not abandoned her. But Mary also left the home for periods of up to half a day at a time, so that others had major responsibility. She located a reliable babysitter and got a neighbor to agree to care for Jenny occasionally. Mr. Henning also continued to provide some of the care whenever he was home. Over a six-month period Jenny changed a great deal. She not only would accept help from others but she would smile and reach out to new people whenever she met them. Mary commented, "It was hard to set it all up and even harder to walk out the door sometimes. But when I look at Jenny and me now, I know it was worth it."

Broadening and extending the caregiving role should begin with the other parent, if possible, and opportunities should be sought, and even created, to involve and acquaint the baby with additional persons whenever possible. This is no less important for the child with disability than for other children; on the contrary, it is more important. *Parents must fight the inclination to pity and protect, which may in the long run rob disabled children of their independence, their self-respect, and much of their potential competence.*

In addition to meeting the challenge of caring for the new baby, the parent of the child with a disability will be responsible for carrying out measures to com—pensate for impairment (such as bowel and bladder function in the child with spina bifida), to assure development (such as exercise of the limbs for the child with cerebral palsy), or to meet unpredictable treatment needs (such as infusion of blood products when the child with hemophilia has a bleed). Some of these needs will be present from birth and will remain throughout life; others will appear, change, or disappear as the child develops. When the new parents take their child home, they should have been prepared with a treatment plan and instruction in the techniques needed to care for the child. Often this preparation has been provided by a treatment team. This is a time when parents should ask all the questions that occur to them and seek explanations for directions and procedures they don't understand. Sometimes professionals talk in jargon or use words new to the parents, and they should be asked to explain if their instructions are unclear. Periodic reevaluation and ongoing consultation from a multidisciplinary team is important for most kinds of disability.

The kinds of professionals who usually make up such a team are mentioned in Chapter Ten. While such a team requires careful coordination (much of it from you, the parent), the point of view and knowledge of each specialist is needed and may be invaluable in treating a certain aspect of disability and in monitoring your child's special pattern of development. More knowledge about the needs of special children is available today than can be mastered and retained by a single individual or within a single profession. Each discipline is a source of expert evaluation and recommendation regarding the child's development; at different points in the child's life, each may also be a source of treatment, training, and on-going consultation. A child diagnosed with cerebral palsy may be having difficulty with feeding because of incoordination in muscles of the face and neck. A speech pathologist may assist by studying the child's mouth movements and recommending a feeding procedure. As a child gets to self-feeding, an occupational therapist may consult about adapting a spoon, cup, or dish. Later these staff persons will begin to deal directly with the child as he participates in his own care. In addition to professionals, parent groups are an important source of practical ideas about how-to-do-it, suggestions for devices and adaptation of equipment, and information about additional helpful resources. Some of the best devices have been created by family or friends, and professionals like OTs (occupational therapists) and PTs (physical therapists) are very happy to receive their ideas.

At home you and your child will begin to develop a routine, and that is useful. Most children thrive on a certain amount of routine and regularity in events such as mealtime, bedtime, and playtime—the patterns about which they begin to build life habits. For example, we all know teenagers (and adults!) who leave a trail of clothes through a house, assuming that someone will pick up after them. Toddlers can be introduced gradually to becoming responsible. Provide a specific spot (low hook in closet) where his coat goes when you come in from outdoors, and go through this sequence consistently with your child so that it becomes a part of the whole procedure of walking into the house. A blind child can do this as well as anyone else, including a moderately retarded child.

Children, of course, need stimulation from people and from the things in their environment. They also need the time and opportunity to explore things on their own. You will want to pay attention to this and to gradually increase the time that the child is on his own and entertaining himself.

As the child begins to grow and develop the capacity to initiate independent activity—to get into things, so to speak—the question of setting limits and discipline will arise. *The basic principle to be followed is that, excluding things that cannot be expected because of specific impairment, the expectations, limits, and discipline of the disabled child should be no different from those for other children.* Paola, age three, and his sister Marie, age five, love to make constructions on the floor, combining building blocks and Lincoln Logs. Paola's braces make it hard to get up and down, so when they are done, he replaces things in their box and stacks them while Marie gathers up those that are scattered and then puts everything in the chest. The children long ago decided this system was fair, and neither will allow the other to do less than his share. Obviously, no persons can or should be expected to do things that are physically or mentally impossible for them. But beyond their specific limitations, there should be no special dispensations for the disabled. The goal is for them to live as fully as possible in the world. *As they grow up, the respect of others and, more importantly, their respect for themselves will be in direct proportion to the extent to which they do as much for themselves as possible.* We do them no favor by indulging our own feelings of compassion and pity and letting them get by with less than they can do because life is "so hard" for them. On the contrary, the feeling of pride that people experience in accomplishing something difficult through effort is a prize denied to them if we don't allow, even expect, them to try.

For the parent of the young child with disability, this translates into setting limits (you can't sleep in your parents' bed, for example), setting expectations (you *will* empty the wastebaskets when it's your turn), and when necessary, using the same methods of discipline as for other children. While you are still learning your child's physical and mental limits, professional consultation can be helpful in setting expectations: Can I expect him to learn to dress himself? Should we expect him to walk (in his own manner) around the block with the family? *The principle here is to ask the child to achieve to the limits of his capabilities, stretching them just a bit. Expect a lot, but not the impossible. Avoid stereotyping your child by treating him as though he is fragile or weak in every area of his being or activity when in reality he may have but a few circumscribed limitations.* Many years ago, a family of our acquaintance insisted that their cerebral palsied daughter do everything the family did, even though she might complain and it sometimes slowed them down. They didn't have much consultation then but did it because it seemed right. They endured a good bit of criticism and "how-could-you-be-so-cruel?" looks. Their daughter is now a charming and self-assured adult who is loyal to the family and still fights a bit with her brothers and sisters.

By no means should this call for limits, expectations, and appropriate discipline for your child be interpreted as a call for harshness. With due respect for the frustrations of childrearing, we would suggest firm good humor as the appropriate approach. In Chapter Seven of this book you will find suggestions about child training techniques. You will also find references to more detailed training manuals under Sources of Additional Information at the end of that chapter. Parent-child training programs, particularly for families who have children with specific problems such as developmental disability, hearing impairment, or vision impairment, are available in many communities if you feel the need for further help.

A natural starting place in setting expectations is in learning self-help skills. The beginning of learning to dress oneself is in helping the person who is dressing you, as by extending the arm for the sleeve. Undressing helps to develop these skills, as does completing part of the job, such as by pulling up the sock. Craig is a three-year-old with mild cerebral palsy. When asked what Craig did to assist with dressing, his mother looked surprised and said that she always did it for him, that he couldn't do anything. It was suggested that he be expected to do parts of the process, little things at first, such as pulling off the sock after Mom had pulled it down over the heel or taking the coat off after Mom had gotten one arm out. She began to think of other ways in which skills could be broken down into parts so that Craig could begin to take some self-responsibility. Dressing and bathing can be exercises in physical development as well as self-help.

Self-help skills can also be logically extended into simple chores, that are their responsibility, which should be part of children's lives by the time they are two or three years old. Dressing and undressing can be related to folding laundered clothes and eventually to helping put them away. Drinking from a cup can be extended to getting a drink and finally to putting clean cups away. Early on, children should have simple chores that are their responsibility, with the expectation that eventually they will do them without prompting, thus learning responsibility as well as work. Four-year-old Bobby is a husky lad who is slow in learning skills because his development is delayed. He can't speak much yet, but he *can* sort dark clothes from light ones, load the washer on mother's directions, unload the dryer when the bell rings (even handling hot clothes gingerly), and fold the towels and underclothing. When he is done he demands some praise, and he has earned it.

The early roots of responsibility lie in self-responsibility. In very young children this is seen in the amount of time they can be left alone, their capacity to entertain and amuse themselves, their ability to initiate their own activities. You may wonder about this emphasis on weighty subjects such as independence and responsibility at this early stage in a child's development. Consider an alternative frequently seen: parents seeking help in getting their *teenager* to be independent and responsible. At that age it is a task of monumental difficulty; it is fixing the leaky roof after it is already raining. Long-range well-being and life satisfaction for your child lie in attending to these important traits beginning in the early stages of his development. Leaving children to initiate their own play will eventually lead to learning to initiate their own work.

Mobility is a matter of importance in your child's total development. Mobility may include being moved about or moving oneself about. Wanda is a brain-damaged child who cannot turn herself over or crawl. Her mother places her in different positions and rooms during the day so that she can get different views of her environment. Sometimes she lies in a Tumbleforms chair watching her mother work in the kitchen or her father work in the garage. Sometimes she is placed by a window where she can see trees or wind chimes outside. Sometimes she is placed on the floor with stimulating toys (such as a monkey playing a drum) just beyond her reach so that she will look up and edge toward the toy. Wanda has become responsive to different situations and is a happier child than one left alone in a crib for long periods.

Self-mobility involves the simple ability to move about in one's environment: to roll over; to learn to walk; to use a walker, braces, or wheelchair if necessary. Mobility is also a matter of familiarity with the territory. This begins with introducing the child to the different rooms of the house, then to the porch or deck or backyard. It may be hard to see how keeping Tanya in one room because it is safe can later in her life lead to an inability to go about her hometown, to use a bus, or drive a car. But the link is there.

Communication is another essential element in your child's development. Parent and child are laying the groundwork for communication as they progress from visual and body contact to the interchange of sounds. An effective means of communicaton must be developed early in a child's life and used regularly. If a disability (blindness, deafness, impairment of the muscles that form speech) interferes with early communication, then alternate ways need to be established in order to develop this necessary link to other persons. The blind child should be stimulated with descriptive language along with the introduction of many things to hear and feel. The deaf child should be stimulated visually with gestures and consistent visual cues. Aaron is a three-year-old who is deaf. When he came into the center, he was communicating energetically with his older brother and parents through signing. They spoke as they signed to him, and it was clear that he was very aware of what was going on around him.

The child who cannot form consistent sounds for words should be provided with pictures and objects which he may learn to associate with words. Jacques has cerebral palsy that involved many muscles of his body, including those involved in speech. When asked if he uses different sounds for different things his mother reported that his frequent cries for attention are followed by "20 questions." Mom must ask, "Do you want this, that, or the other?" A way to increase a child's feeling of control over his environment in this case would be to devise a simple language system involving pictures of activities or objects, which can cue a parent about the child's needs. These could include needs such as a cup for a drink of water or a potty-chair for toileting. Janet, with severe cerebral palsy, can indicate that she wants to listen to her tapes by touching the picture of a tape recorder. In this way she feels some control and responsibility for herself and feels she can be understood, even at a simple level. *Any child needs an early basic method by which he can display wants and needs and can understand his parents' communications.* A useful by-product of this is a decrease in the amount of frustrating time spent by parents in trying to interpret the child's attempts at wordless communication. The child who appears to be fussy, for example, may be attempting to communicate something. When he is not understood, he may go on to a tantrum. This may disappear after he learns a better way to communicate or when the parents learn to interpret his message.

Socialization will be important to your child's enjoyment of life, and social skills will have a great deal to do with the quality of his acceptance by others. Socialization begins when you and the child coo at each other. After a while it includes the other parent, adult relatives, and friends. Interestingly, many children with disabilities have far more experience and skill in dealing with adults than they do in dealing with persons of their age, their peers. Some children have had many hospitalizations and because of this have had more contact with adults and have learned ways of relating to them. At the same time this has caused less contact with peers and the opportunities for peer interaction. Difficulty in dealing with peers is a problem that appears to feed upon and magnify itself. If you're uncomfortable with peers you stay away from them; thus you don't get the practice that would increase your skills, and so you stay away some more. For this reason socialization with peers is another area best dealt with early in life. It should begin in the form of play with (or beside) brothers and sisters, if any. Similar-aged neighbor children should be included. Make an effort to get to know them and to invite them to play if it doesn't happen naturally. It may include time spent visiting cousins or in religious school. Provide toys, equipment, or settings that lend themselves to activities that can be shared by disabled and nondisabled alike. Such play needs remote supervision by adults, applied as lightly and infrequently as circumstances permit, to prevent bodily harm but not to iron out minor differences.

As your child approaches three you should investigate the availability of nursery school or preschool facilities. Headstart (a federally subsidized program for disadvantaged children) is available in many communities and has a specific mandate to provide services to a certain percentage of children with disabling conditions. The school you choose should be able and willing to accommodate the special needs of your child by adapting activities and providing any special care that may be required. In many instances, children with disability can be accommodated in regular classes at the preschool level. In accord with our principle, they should be expected to do all within their capacity, but not the impossible. The classrooms for children with disabilities may have the advantage of specially trained teachers and special equipment. Some children may require this for effective participation. The advantage of special teachers and facilities must be balanced against the experience of dealing with the broad spectrum of children in the mainstream situation. In general, the mainstream will be the most desirable alternative if your child can participate effectively in that setting, but not if it means he will spend a large portion of his time sidelined.

Enrollment in some preschool setting is strongly encouraged for the following reasons: 1) the socialization with peers; 2) the enriched stimulation and learning it affords, as well as the opportunity to learn the skills (such as sitting at a desk, being quiet on request) needed for school participation; and 3) the respite it gives parents, who need to maintain a balanced life of their own if they are to be of maximum benefit to their children.

4

OFF TO SCHOOL
Ages Six Through Twelve

In the charming terminology of the Old South, your child has gone from being a lap-baby to a yard-baby and is now ready to become a school-baby. Going off to school has traditionally played an important role in the growing independence of the child. With leaving the home for school we frequently find separation anxiety, which can be as difficult for Mom (or Dad) as for the youngster. Hopefully this adjustment to kindergarten or first grade will be based on previous experience in nursery or pre-school, allowing parents and child to be brave and confident as the child goes off to handle this new adventure.

The first day of school is one that calls for skill and restraint on the part of Mom and Dad. You will need to assure yourself that the child has arrived at the right place and is in responsible hands. You will need to give her enough support, by your presence and measured (not effusive) reassurance, to give her confidence in entering the situation. Your job then becomes one of making a graceful and timely exit—about as much farewell as if you were leaving him with Grandma or the neighbor, no exaggerated display of emotion and no sudden returns to see if everything is all right! The teacher has been through this before and may give you helpful cues. You should have confidence in the child, in the teacher, and in the arrangements that you made in advance with the school personnel.

A good deal of thought, planning, and prearrangement should have taken place before that first day of school for a child with a disability. You should begin this by obtaining the advice and recommendations of the people who have been serving her—the treatment team and the teachers from the preschool setting. You should try to make their recommendations about the child's needs available to the school authorities at least several months in advance of the time she is to enter a public school program. A word of caution here: in enrolling a child with special school needs, it will be important for the contact and the planning to be done with the participation of the special education or other program specialists in your school district. Simply enrolling in the nearest elementary school without informing them of the child's special needs will not be enough and may well result in confusion, conflict, and time lost in getting the right program and appropriate services.

The issues to be considered in advance are those related to the kind and amount of the resources that your child will need to get the most benefit from the school experience. Do medical and physical needs mean that special treatment procedures, facilities, or personnel will be required during the school day? Is special transportation needed? Can your child function, from an educational and a social point of view, in a regular classroom? Is a special classroom needed? If your child is in a wheelchair, are the school, its classrooms, and its restrooms accessible? Are special modes of instruction needed, such as the use of manual sign, Braille, or language boards? Will home tutoring be required as part of the service? Or a program that combines several of these elements?

These program questions need to be considered in advance, and the process begins with the appropriate school personnel getting a good idea of your child's special strengths, disabilities, and needs. The more that is known in advance, the more likely it is that your child will begin with the services she needs. It should be pointed out, however, that these decisions and arrangements need not be written in stone and that parents, teachers, and (hopefully) children should keep an open mind about making changes based on experience. Soon after your child has started school, the particular combination of needs and the services she requires should be written into a formal Individualized Educational Program (IEP). You should expect to be included in the planning of this program, as you will be asked to give it final approval.

Communication between you and school can rarely be overdone! Teachers are many things: usually effective, usually busy, usually interested in your child. Mr. and Mrs. Winkosky had gone to school the week before opening especially to tell the teacher that George would be wearing new hearing aids when he started second grade. They asked the teacher to let them know whether George was in fact wearing them in class (George would rather not). They also wanted to know how well the aids were working; could he hear the teacher? They waited patiently for several weeks, then impatiently for several more. After three months they called the school. Lo and behold, George had been assigned to the classroom of Miss Gregory, not to the classroom of Mrs. Aletis! Their careful discussion with Mrs. Aletis had gone for naught. Miss Gregory was pleased to meet them, and things worked fine for the rest of the year. George did need to have his aids adjusted several times that year. Nothing gets accomplished by staying home in silence wondering, What in the world do they think they're doing? Many questions and problems can be solved by asking about them or offering information. Begin with the assumption that the teacher is sincere, competent, and trying to do it right. You will probably find that to be the case. Establish contact and let the teacher know how to get in touch with you.

Sometimes, after a period of constructive dialogue and attempts to jointly solve a problem with the teacher, you may find yourself with an honest difference of opinion. That is the time to carry your question to the supervisors of the specialized program that serves your child, as well as to the principal. Your effectiveness as an advocate will be increased by the knowledge and the confidence in your opinion that you developed by having the prior discussion with the teacher.

Sometimes teachers or school administrators can be less than sensitive to parents' understanding of school problems. They fall into educationese-style jargon. This creates the same difficulty as medical jargon, and parents should be persistent about asking for clarification and about having their own questions addressed. Also, educators may center their attention on administrative details without including the parents in relevant discussions. At a meeting regarding Jim, a student with vision and motor problems, typing lessons were recommended. Jim's mother looked lost as the school personnel launched into a long discussion of how this would fit into Jim's schedule, who had the budget for the service, and which teacher would be responsible for it. The school psychologist interrupted to tell the mother that typing was suggested because of Jim's laborious handwriting and that it had nothing to do with the long-term prospects for his ability to see. Relief flooded into Mother's face! Her biggest worry was that Jim might totally lose his vision. She had been overcome by this deluge of talk on top of her preoccupation and worry. They had essentially excluded her from the discussion by talking in language that she could not penetrate and had failed to notice that their main concern was not the mother's main concern.

As your child approaches and enters the school years, differences between her and the other children may become more evident. These differences increase as the child gets older; the fact that an infant doesn't roll over at the same age as others is less apparent to others than the fact that a three-year-old is not able to walk or a four-year-old is not able to talk. If your child's *rate* of development of motor, speech, or mental skills is delayed, this difference can be analyzed in another way. Suppose, for example, she is developing in certain abilities at only three-quarters the rate of other children. The difference at age four will be one year; the others will be speaking in longer sentences and be better coordinated. The difference at age twelve will be three years; she will barely be able to read, while the others are reading quite competently. As significant differences in ability become noticeable to the child and others, this can become the focus of important feelings and social attitudes, both positive and negative. These differences often become obvious on entry to school, when children are typically grouped by age. There are some things that can help your child in handling these feelings and attitudes, and they include knowledge of her disability and its meaning and awareness of her own areas of strength and competence.

Talking about the disability is important. It should not be the focus of every discussion with or about the child, but neither should it be a forbidden topic. Discussion should be factually accurate, matter-of-fact in tone, and at the child's level of understanding. The child should have a name for her disability so long as it does not carry the burden of a negative stereotype. The child should also have a simple explanation of the disability. For cerebral palsy or spina bifida it may be "It means I can't walk." For diabetes or cystic fibrosis, "It means I must take medicine and follow a special diet." Where there is a negative stereotype, as in mental retardation, the explanation may replace the name, as in "It means I need special help in school." It is inevitable that the child (and you) will be confronted with situations which are handled best with a simple, nondetailed explanation, and if the disability has been discussed occasionally and casually at home with brothers and sisters, friends, and relatives, your comfort and competence in handling the situation will be increased. Disability should be discussed when it is relevant to the topic at hand. For example, if the family is planning a hike, then whether Johnny will be included should be discussed in terms of his ability to walk the distance. If the plan is for a family game, then it should be discussed in terms of what role Sue can play: might she be scorekeeper, have someone run the bases for her, or play Ping-Pong from her wheelchair with no modifications needed.

The infusion of a sense of humor in the discussion

of disability is worthwhile, so that eventually Johnny can accept (or better yet, participate in) gentle joking about his incapacity. For example, on setting out for a walk you might say, "Let's go, Hopalong" or "Roll 'em, hot wheels!" To be able to joke with your child about disability says a great deal about the security each of you feels. It also means that he is on his way to developing a perspective on himself and a social skill that will stand him in good stead all of his life. Big cautionary note: this does not condone cruel teasing or scapegoating by anyone. Your fondness should always show through. Your child will eventually meet bullying or meanness in the world, and he doesn't need it from "friends" or relatives.

There are no foolproof methods for dealing with teasing. Sometimes it can be ignored, but not always; teasers can be persistent and intrusive. Sometimes it can be handled with a humorous rejoinder such as one used by a child of our acquaintance, "I got hit by a cement truck; what's your excuse?" The support of friends can help in handling the sting of teasing by showing that there are people who prefer to be with *him* and by providing consensus that the bully's opinion is not shared by the whole world. Sometimes teasing is just plain humiliating, uncomfortable, and inescapable. You should hear out your child's anger and frustration when he comes home from such an episode. Later he may need to be quietly reminded that there are others around who respect him and who do not tease him cruelly. Prolonged and persistent teasing or scapegoating may call for intervention by parents or authorities. This is an approach that should be used sparingly but not ruled out.

As you can see, talking about things is helpful. Conversations with your child will help her to learn to talk about what is on her mind, whether it be about the kids in school, the bus ride home, or how she felt during an exchange with her teacher. Children become better communicators with practice. By contrast, if they do not have opportunities for expression or are ignored or criticized when they do talk, they hesitate to venture into conversations.

One way that you can promote talking is by being a good listener. Sometime during the day you should make a point of checking in with your child and listening to her talk about what is going on in her life or whatever she may choose to talk about. Arrival home from school is a good time for this if you can do it. You should practice at listening. Give occasional short responses that let her know you hear and understand. Phrases like "That must have been fun," "Oh, wow," "What a bummer!" or just "Uh-huh" will let her know you are tuned in. Sometimes short questions may be appropriate, especially ones that respond to what you have heard, such as "What did your team make for the exhibit?" or "Who was there?" Your goal should be to hear a general description of the child's day, including good and bad experiences, and not an accounting or an inflated recitation of accomplishments. If you find yourself conducting a drawn-out question-and-answer quiz, however, drop it; better to share a quiet time together than an interrogation.

If you work at establishing a listening time, eventually your child will come to expect it, and dialogue should flow fairly easily. Such shared time will strengthen your relationship and help to minimize the communication problems that seem to develop a little later as the teen years approach. Talking to you at some length will also have the effect of increasing your child's ability to put things into words and to formulate opinions about the events in her life.

Another way to promote talking is by not answering *for* your child. Cheryl was having some difficulty with her new leg braces. When the therapist asked her to explain the problem, Mom interrupted and talked for her. She clearly and quickly defined the problem. Cheryl sat quietly as she was discussed. Her mother unwittingly denied her the experience of explaining her own problem and also the experience of learning how to talk to the therapist. After this was pointed out to Mom (on the side), she began to let Cheryl answer questions and to provide elaboration only when necessary. Cheryl began to feel more responsibility for helping to solve problems as they came along.

Everyone needs to be good at something, whether it be raising goldfish or playing chess, drawing pictures or cleaning a room, remembering facts or playing ball. Among the many things your child *can* do, some will stick out, and they are his strengths. Find these strengths and help him build them and praise him for them realistically. (Overdramatic, exaggerated praise comes off sounding phony, and eventually he'll discount it.) Strengths might lie in school abilities like arithmetic or hobbies like beading belts or social skills like making people feel relaxed or community activities like helping in Sunday school. These are the foundation on which we build our self-esteem. These are also the competencies on which we build our eventual social and vocational skills. Remember, we don't have to be Nobel Prize winners or astronauts to have self-esteem; bookkeepers and janitors and mechanics have pride in their work— and your child can, too. Eventually he should be thinking, "Well, I can't do *that* (play hockey) but I sure can do *this* (talk, sell, entertain)."

Self-esteem based on feeling competent in certain areas is an important part of self-concept, but not all of it. Self-concept is the way we view our total selves. It takes into account our strengths and our weaknesses, our virtues and our foibles, our beauty marks and our warts. It is based on our knowledge of self. We each observe ourselves in action, noting successes and failures and evaluating the results of our efforts. *The most important source of our self-knowledge, however, is what other people tell us about ourselves.* This is done through large numbers of clues over long periods of time. Sometimes it is the direct statement "That was great" or "That was lousy." More often it is the subtle message sent by the quirk of an eyebrow, the frown, the lack of enthusiasm, the laugh, the spontaneous delight. *It is essential for all of us that, over time, we come to a self-appraisal that is realistic enough to allow us to understand how others see us and to set goals for ourselves that we have a reasonable chance of meeting successfully. In order to arrive at a realistic self-appraisal, it is necessary that the disabled child get feedback from others that is reasonably honest and accurate.*

Perry's father had always wanted to be a professional baseball player but never got beyond a brief trial in the minor leagues. When Perry was born with cerebral palsy, his dad decided that that should not stand in Perry's way. He coached him in the backyard and Perry spent endless hours practicing hitting, catching, and throwing. He had trouble with coordinating his hands and eyes but gradually learned to hit the ball. He could get it in from center field, although his throw was a little weak. Dad said he would be on his way to the big leagues if he kept trying. At eight Perry joined a Little League team. The coach didn't agree with the opinions that Dad put forth all the time, but the coach kept quiet and had Perry play at least a little in every game. Perry occasionally made a base hit and usually was able to cover center field. Dad complained at home that the coach was not giving Perry enough playing time, considering his big league potential. At twelve Perry went out for the city Babe Ruth League team, confident he would succeed. He was not chosen. Dad complained, and Perry was given a uniform and allowed to sit on the bench. During practice Perry was not able to keep up and couldn't hit against the fast pitching. Eventually he concluded for himself that he was a failure. He decided it was his fault. He hadn't worked hard enough. Perry, who had achieved a degree of baseball competence that was *remarkable* for his level of physical strength and coordination, concluded that he was a personal failure and it was his own responsibility. He gave up baseball entirely. He withdrew. It took him three years, some help from a counselor, and the development of a new set of skills and hobbies (backpacking, cross-country skiing, computer programming) before he began to see himself once more as a competent and worthwhile person.

The matter of appropriate feedback for a child with significant disability can be difficult to achieve; it requires a sensitive balance. That child (like all of us) needs hope, needs some light at the end of the tunnel. That is the reason finding strengths and encouraging them is important. On the other hand, if praise is regularly exaggerated and the child is protected from ordinary participation and feedback, he may arrive at a false and inflated assessment of his abilities, one that may lead to heartbreak and disillusion when he tests it against reality.

There are some principles that may help in this matter of balancing praise and encouragement with a realistic assessment of the child's skills and of the demands of the world. For one thing, praise should be tempered, should not be over-extravagant, and especially should not be generalized to other situations in ways that are unwarranted. When the kid hits a good one with the whiffle bat, say "Wow, that's great," not "Wow, next year you'll be ready for Little League." (Unless you honestly think he will be ready.) If the kid sets his heart on the Little League team and you think he won't make it, say "Well, you sure can try. That's pretty tough competition." (Not "no", but not "yes.") Then try to move him gradually into more challenges (playing with a league ball, perhaps) so he can begin to make his own judgments. You may even change your opinion. In general, a flat "No, you won't be able to do it" will be too deflating and also may close off options that could turn out to be possible. On the other hand, a "yes" you know is grossly unrealistic will set up false expectations and future hurts. In the end, he will need to learn to make those judgments for himself.

During the school years and later in life, your child will have opportunities to join in social and recreational activities with other disabled persons. For some, the decision to participate in such groups is an easy and natural one. For others, usually those concerned with the stigma of disability, it is difficult. There are some criteria that can be useful in making this decision about participating in the world of the disabled in addition to participating in the mainstream. For example, in mainstream participation can the child experience real peer competition? Can he win sometimes? Does social participation include getting some genuine acceptance and developing at least a few close friends? These issues are discussed further in Chapter Eleven.

Our observation is that the disabled children (and adults) who do best move in and out of both worlds, the world of the disabled and the mainstream. This does *not* mean that the child must socialize or find recreation primarily with other disabled persons. Such experiences can be quite limited or they can be extensive, according to the needs and the desires of the child. Experiences with disabled persons can be enriching to the life of every child, with or without disability. If you have nondisabled children, they will profit from some participation along with their disabled brother or sister.

Opportunities for experience in group activities with other disabled children will begin to present themselves during the preteen school years. Some opportunities are in the school or in the form of extended school programs. Some are in activities such as the Special Olympics, recreational programs in the city parks, and camps for persons with a variety of disabilities. Annual participation in a summer camp is a highly desirable part of your child's development of independence and self-responsibility skills. This may be a mainstream experience in a Y, Scout, church, or other kind of camp, or it may be in a special camp for the disabled. Some children participate in both. Here again, you should use the criteria mentioned earlier regarding peer competition, social acceptance, and learning to decide which experiences will be best for your child. Special note: camping with the family is a good idea, too, but it isn't a substitute for the experience of being with peers away from parents.

*   *   *

The time of these early school years represents another critical era in the climb toward independence. The main principle remains: *Never do for the disabled child what she can do for herself.* This particularly includes all aspects of self-care such as dressing (including choice of clothes), bathing, making her bed, and cleaning her room. By now the child should have additional regular chores, such as setting or clearing the table, emptying the wastebaskets, feeding pets, or helping in the garden. Part of the responsibility should include initiating the chore. The child should also be learning simple food preparation, such as getting things from the refrigerator and fixing a sandwich.

In developing self-help skills in the child, it is important to avoid, wherever possible, deciding that it is easier to do it yourself than to wait for the child to do it. The result of doing it yourself is that the child does not get the practice that would increase her skill and speed. This comes up often in the areas of bathing and dressing. Again, no one should be asked to do what is impossible. It may take a long time to learn how to dress, and some persons may always require partial assistance (in putting on trousers or tying shoes, for example). When these limits have been established, the child should be expected to do all that is within her capacity. This may require getting up early, but that is more desirable than failing to develop and polish these skills, which are so important to self-image as well as to independence.

Gradually increasing periods of self-responsibility are also part of the climb toward independence. This begins with time alone in a room, the yard, or some other part of the house. It also includes visits away from home in the daytime, perhaps to neighbors and friends, and overnight visits, beginning with relatives but also extending to friends. Your child needs to become comfortable with being alone or with others, up to the limit of her capacity.

Another area of responsibility that directly affects your child's capacity to be alone or in the company of others revolves about her knowledge of her disability. She should be aware of any treatments or medications that are required, when they're needed, and how they are carried out. She should participate in setting up and carrying out home treatment as is appropriate to her age and understanding. She should be given the responsibility for preventive care, such as regularly shifting body weight in a wheelchair to prevent skin irritation and pressure sores. If lack of cleanliness and careful personal hygiene results in offensive odors, the child should be made aware of this. She should also learn the relationship between prohibited activities (breaking diet, playing contact sports, skipping medications) and the pain or illness which follows. It should be clear that the responsibility lies with her, and it will be desirable for the child to experience some minor discomfort as the result of such misbehaviors rather than always preventing any negative consequences through the parent playing dictator, policeman, and guard. Thus she will begin to see that the prohibited activity has negative consequences and that the choice is under her control. *It is extremely important that there be a gradual but successful transition in this focus of responsibility from others to self during the preteen years.*

5

GROWING UP
The Teen Years

You remember the teen years—when your body grew in strange and wondrous ways, when you looked in the mirror and wondered who could love you, when your mood could be changed from despair to euphoria by a phone call, and when your parents couldn't possibly understand the feelings and opinions you shared with your friends. You can expect much the same with your child. Disability does not mean that the body and the hormones and the social needs do not develop. If your child is growing toward independence, he will have the same need as others to establish an identity, a being, and a set of attitudes and opinions separate from his parents'. While in some cases children with a disability may, by virtue of limited experience, be delayed in entering the adolescent social experience, you should nevertheless look forward to adolescence as a period of bitter-sweet pleasure for your child and as a necessity if he is to become an independent adult.

It is an interesting irony that in this time when he is establishing separateness from his parents it becomes important to the teen to be just like his peers. The social approval of his peer group is necessary if he is to experiment with being different from (independent of) his parents. He needs peer support to tell him he is not alone. The disabled teen is subject to all the stresses of the nondisabled, with a few additional ones. He may be close to his parents, recognize his dependence on them, and appreciate them more than most teens, so that even temporary loss of their approval (perhaps for dyeing his hair orange) can be threatening and make it difficult for him to fully join the teen group. If his experiences have been restricted to parents and older family members, he may have a patronizing "little adult" outlook which will not help him get along with peers. Rebellion can be harder for him because of fear of loss of his parents' approval. Even more to the point, at an age when conformity to the peer group is important and when fellow teens have not developed some of the insight and compassion of maturity, he may find himself systematically excluded because of differentness in appearance, walk, or talk. Such exclusion may be related to superficial appearances, to disability that is limiting only in certain activities, or to disability that broadly limits the teen's capacity to share in the social, recreational, or intellectual life of the teen group. A judgment about which of these is the case should help in deciding whether to focus his efforts on doing everything like everyone else, choosing only a limited number of activities in the mainstream (as most people ordinarily do), or seeking activities that have been especially adapted to the needs of youths with handicaps.

It will be useful if you can help your teen understand the wisdom most of us arrive at sometime in life: the knowledge that being liked by everyone isn't necessary. We need a few friends who know us well, like us for our unique qualities, and share some of our interests. We do not have to belong to the coolest social group on campus or be close friends with the class president or the football hero. Most of all, we don't need to be accepted by everyone! The world contains some people who value only qualities we will never have, such as the ability to sing opera or pole-vault; it contains others who are hopelessly prejudiced against everyone who is "different." We need to coexist with them all, but we don't need their endorsement. We do need our own small support group, and from the teen years on, it should include more than our parents.

In finding the social and recreational niches which are right for him, it will be important that your teen be aware of and feel confidence in his areas of strength and competence besides having a general idea of his limitations. A large degree of his sense of competence will come from the skills he has learned at home in taking care of himself and being independent, developing an *I can do it for myself* attitude.

The self-help and independence skills started early in life need special honing and refining in the teen years. Think of your home as the training ground for your teen to learn the skills she will need in order to live independently in the future. The school may supplement with some home economics, personal finance, automobile maintenance, or home repair training, but rarely do these courses cover everything needed, and there is no guarantee that your teen will personally learn all the skills offered. Besides, they won't teach the recipe for Mom's own hamburger stew or how to dry clothes in a bathroom. It is useful to start by assuming that your teen will be living alone or with a peer roommate in an apartment. Many adults with disabilities do live on their own. What skills do they need? Even if you think your teen will not attain that level of independent living, how many of those skills *can* she learn?

Most of the necessary independence skills can be seen as extensions of the self-help skills your teen has already been developing. They should be expanded to every aspect of daily living that is within her physical and mental grasp. She began by learning to dress herself, making her own choices of clothing according to the weather and the day's activities. She has learned to fold and put away clothing and now must learn how to operate a washer (including choice of detergent, bleach, softener) and dryer. She should be involved in shopping for clothing, making choices for herself that consider style, quality, and cost.

She began by learning how to feed herself, to get a drink of water, and to get simple foods from the refrigerator. She needs to learn how to make a sandwich, heat soup, make tea or hot chocolate, cook a roast, toss a salad, bake a cake. She should learn to use appliances such as stove, dishwasher, and mixer. You and she together may figure out how to adapt utensils to her grip and hand strength or what kind of stove she can operate most easily. (Stoves with controls up front rather than set back are usually best.) Living independently will also involve the ability to plan a menu and shop in the food market, taking advantage of the advertised specials. Eating, of course, is not only a physical necessity but a social skill; consider the date, the dinner party, and lunch in the company cafeteria. Your teen should be acquiring experience in eating in public places such as restaurants, choosing from the menu, and negotiating the cafeteria line. Perhaps this is the time to make another important point: *Growing up as an independent person who happens to have a disability also involves knowing when you need help and being willing and able to ask for it in a way that is polite but not self-demeaning.* Cafeteria lines can be a useful and interesting place for learning. Because the physically handicapped person often needs help, it is a good place to practice asking for it in a matter-of-fact way. It should be polite ("Please" and then "Thank you" are in order) but without apology or a feeling of guilt. Do keep it polite, however. That a person has a disability does not mean strangers or friends owe him help without a word of thanks.

Because someone is receiving help, it is not unusual for the cafeteria line worker to assume that the person is mentally incompetent and to ask the helper what the disabled person would like to order. By no means should the helping person respond to such a question. In that way it can become a learning experience for the cafeteria worker as well. Two of our friends taught a poor cafeteria worker who made this mistake. They decided that she was treating Ted in the wheelchair like a creature from outer space, so they developed a scheme to carry on an elaborate conversation in gibberish when she asked Tom what "he" (pointing to Ted) wanted. After an extended exchange of nonsense syllables, Tom would say "a hamburger" or "soup" (a decision they had made in advance). Over several days, the cafeteria worker became mystified, then inquisitive, then embarrassed, and finally a very attentive friend of Ted's, even after he offered to teach her "the language."

Your teen's mobility began long ago with rolling over, crawling, and eventually learning how to get around by walking or using aids such as crutches, walker, or wheelchair. She should have learned her way around the neighborhood and how to get to school and back. She has been going places with parents and other adults. She now needs to learn to get about the community on her own. This may begin with riding the city bus, learning to use it at first with someone else, and one transfer at a time, if necessary. It may involve the use of special transportation for the handicapped; if that is necessary, she should learn how to call to make her own arrangements. An important part of your teen's vocational future will depend upon whether she can get to the job, how long it takes, and how much it costs to get there.

Driving a car is of great symbolic and considerable practical importance to the American teen. It makes the teen crazy to do it and the parent crazy deciding if he should be allowed to. Driving involves three major factors: 1) the mental capacity to understand the procedure, follow routes and signs, and apply judgment under stress; 2) the physical strength and coordination to operate the vehicle; and 3) sufficiently rapid physical and mental reaction time. Consideration also needs to be given to vision and to the possibility of uncontrolled seizures. Great strides have been made in adapting vehicles so that requirements of physical strength and, to some extent, coordination have been minimized.

Our position is that every teen, with or without a disability, who believes he is capable of learning to drive a car deserves the opportunity to find himself sitting in the middle of a large, paved, flat, empty area behind the wheel of a suitably equipped or modified car with a capable driving instructor who will work hard to help him succeed. Let the experience speak for itself! We know that a large number of disabled persons *can* drive. We know that a large number can't. We know that it's hard to accept a flat "no" without trying, and so we advise a trial if it seems remotely possible. The driver with a disability should have the same preparation for driving as others, including classroom training and testing of his proficiency. Specialized evaluation and driver training may be available through rehabilitation centers or similar community agencies. Independence in driving should be approached in stages: first with an experienced driver: then alone on short daytime trips in familiar territory, and so on, increasing in difficulty and responsibility. At the expense of drawing the ire of the teenagers who, we hope, will be reading this with their parents, we should also add that there may be times when waiting a few years beyond the minimum driving age will be helpful in attaining the physical or social maturity required for competent driving.

Learning to drive will often mark the beginning of great strides in personal independence as well as in social and recreational participation on the part of the disabled teen. If it is within the teen's capacity, it is well worth the effort to obtain the appropriate vehicle and training and worth the white knuckles and nervous waits it will cost the parent. Once you have determined that your teenager has the qualifications for driving and a vehicle she can handle, she should receive leeway to try her independence as much as any other teen. She should also get equal discipline if she acts foolishly. But avoid the temptation to use one error to write off the whole idea as a mistake.

Certain aspects of development during the teen years should be directed specifically toward increasing responsibility. For example, thcrc should be substantial chores, and the teen should be expected to do them without prompting; this should be introduced in the beginning as part of the chore.

Another opportunity for responsibility development may involve the matter of waking and getting up in the morning, which can be an exasperating matter if it remains the responsibility of the parent. The solution to this is a personal alarm clock as soon as the teen is old enough to learn how to set it himself. This may call for some real fortitude on the part of the parent when the teen fails to get up on his own. When that happens he should suffer some natural consequences for not getting up, such as having to skip breakfast, having to make up schoolwork at a time that he could otherwise use for recreation, and particularly, having to personally explain tardiness or absence to the teacher. If the parent can hold out through one or two such episodes, the problem is usually self-correcting.

By the teen years the disabled person should have a thorough knowledge of the nature of his disability, of the limitations (in activities and diet for example) it imposes, and the treatment it requires. The responsibility for observing those limitations should be his, not his parents'. He should participate in and probably carry out most of his own treatments. Many become more skillful (and braver) than their parents in doing so. Many teenagers with hemophilia infuse their own blood products at home. The teen should be responsible for knowing when treatments, such as percussing in cystic fibrosis, are needed and how they are carried out. He should be responsible for care of his own appliances, as in changing his hearing-aid batteries or noting when wheelchair repair is needed.

A particular area for concern is personal hygiene. Where the disability includes difficulties with bowel and bladder control, such as is often the case with spina bifida, accidents or lack of cleanliness can easily result in offensive odors. What's more, it is easy for the disabled person to accommodate to them so that he no longer notices the smell. He needs to learn that the odor is offensive to others and that they will avoid him if he smells. Fairness or social nicety has nothing to do with it; he will be ostracized, and even worse, likely be belittled by others. Manny became embarrassed about "how I used to smell" after he learned to keep himself clean and then began to notice odors from some of his friends. He became the scourge of his teenage group, with no hesitation about saying, "Man, you stink!" Amazingly, most of his friendships were strengthened by this behavior, and the group atmosphere was certainly improved. The teen should know the precautions that will help to avoid accidents and the measures that are necessary to clean up when they occur. Being aware of the problem and doing something about it should be totally his responsibility. Anyone who is his friend should tell him when he needs to take action.

We have written at length and in serious terms about self-help skills and responsibility because we believe they are critically important. No one else is likely to assume the responsibility for teaching them to your child, and no one else could do it as well. You can't leave it to schools or workshops. Having these skills will add enormously to your teen's sense of competence. Not being able to care for herself to the level of her capacity can have some important negative consequences. People are usually quite generous in providing others with help that they obviously need. They *may* provide help to those who need or ask for it but appear to be capable of doing more for themselves. In the latter case it is likely to be done grudgingly. *The matter of helping oneself to the limits of capacity becomes a matter of the respect of others as well as a matter of self-respect.* It can represent the difference between a life that is satisfying or not. Let us also say that teaching and growing up with a young person can be fun. Teaching cooking can be fun, even if the first request is how to make pizza! Shopping for clothes with a teen can be fun, even if the T-shirts purchased are tie-dyed or say ELECTRIC BANANAS on the back. Some of the best fun of all will eventually come from sharing experiences with the independent young adult who emerges from this process.

Just as your home is the training ground for self-help skills, so it is also the training ground for attitudes toward disability. Does the young person learn to look at herself as someone to be cared for and pitied, or does she look at herself pragmatically, as someone with a problem who has the capacity to work out a method of caring for herself? The approach that is used in the home will shape the way the individual sees herself. An unrestrained attitude of pity will lead her to look at herself as a pitiful person. When it is assumed that a person cannot, or should not, do things without help, she will come to look at herself (and other handicapped persons) as helpless. Similarly, overzealous attempts to hide or deny the handicap will suggest that it is unacceptable or something to be ashamed of. Parents and siblings should look upon themselves as models for the person with the handicap, as well as models for relatives, neighbors, and friends, in showing respect for the competence and responsibility of persons with disabilities.

                        ⋆   ⋆   ⋆

At the high-school level there will be choices about schooling that parallel those made in the beginning and throughout the school years. Can your teen function physically and socially in mainstream courses and profit from them? Should part of her time be spent in a special program or resource room, with adapted approaches and content tailored to her needs? Strengths and weaknesses take on a double meaning now. There should be continued efforts to build up areas of deficiency (basic reading or math skills, for example). But now there should also be a concerted effort to develop methods that supplement or compensate for those areas of weakness. Bob with the reading problem may be encouraged to learn by listening, through lectures or tapes; Lisa with the math problem may be taught to carry and use a small calculator to make change. Efforts should also be made to develop strengths. Larry with art or mechanical talents should be encouraged to spend time to develop them fully; Sarah with skills in writing, speaking, or persuading others should be facilitated in using them. The fact that deficiencies remain in *some* areas should not be used as a reason to prevent full development and expression in other areas of strength.

Sometimes determination and an ingratiating grin can make a big difference. I knew Tony Falcon from the spina bifida clinic, where we helped him with school and career planning. He requires a wheelchair for mobility. We knew he attended our son's high school, which is on two floors and has no passenger elevator. When we wondered about this, Tony replied, "No problem. I just wait at the foot or the head of the stairs until the first four guys come along, and they carry me up or down." When we asked our son he said, "Oh, Tony. He must have nerves of steel! We carry him around every which

way, and he just sits there and cracks jokes." Tony
obviously has a strength in interpersonal skills (as well
as nerves of steel!).

The high school years also involves another choice
point which cannot be ignored, and that the young
person who plans to go on to a four-year college. A
four-year college degree is often highly desirable for a
person with a disability who has the necessary ability
and the academic interest. It is also highly desired by
many families. Hank was born with mild cerebral palsy,
which caused weakness in his left arm and leg. In his
case it also caused some slowness in mental functioning
and some trouble in organizing complicated thoughts.
His tested ability was low average. Hank's dad was an
architect and his older sister a sophomore at the state
university. Hank was a junior in high school who had
always said he would be "an architect like Dad." The
family encouraged him because they thought college
was a good idea for everyone, and the high school counselor said nothing, even though they all knew that Hank
was not an especially good scholar. In fact, he made a C
average by virtue of studying several hours every night
and taking easy track courses such as personal finance
for math and general science instead of chemistry or
physics. His written essays were just fair, but the teacher
felt that this was because of his difficulty in handwriting, so she gave him C's or B's. Hank was a personable
fellow, and no one wanted to be unpleasant to him. In an
extended career counseling interview, Hank came close
to tears and finally confided that he *knew* that he
couldn't do college work but that he could not tell his
parents because they would be so disappointed and
"everyone" thought he could do it. In a careful interview

with the parents, they were able to say that they believed Hank could not do college work but didn't want to damage his self-concept or deny him an opportunity. Eventually it was possible to discuss the matter with Hank and his parents together. The upshot was that a plan was formulated in which Hank attended a community college where he learned food service and restaurant-operation skills and took some basic management courses, including business English, business law, and bookkeeping. He went on to function successfully, rising to assistant manager in a restaurant.

Hank's story had a happier ending than many which are similar. In other cases, a teen similar to Hank has become convinced that he *will* go to college, and his parents do not want to hear otherwise. The resolution then is often a series of unsuccessful attempts at college, with feelings of frustration and failure and anger. A great deal of time is lost in the process, and an even greater amount of time must go by before the person begins to feel competent in a job or other activities that are suited to his abilities.

The teen who wants to go to four-year college should take upper-level math and English as well as other college preparatory courses in science and social studies. Parents and school counselors who encourage or just go along with college plans should see that the teen is advised to take such courses and is enrolled in them. Parents and school counselors who find themselves unable or unwilling to advise such a teen to enroll in college preparatory courses should question the usefulness of the feedback they are giving by seeming to endorse a college plan. It may be that the teen has an important need to modify her aspirations by hearing the suggestion that there are other goals and other training places (such as a community college) that might also be considered. Again, the approach should not be one of flat "No!" but rather "Maybe, but there are also other possibilities..." and the suggestion of alternatives. A "yes" should be accompanied by advice about the things the teen needs to do and the courses she needs to take to prepare herself to function in a four-year college setting.

Planning for college *or* planning a high school program that emphasizes vocational rather than academic training may mean that vocational evaluation and career counseling are needed early in the high school years so that the school program can be matched to the future goal. For further discussion of this point, see Chapter Thirteen.

Your teen will carry her capacity for independence and responsibility, and her feelings of competence, into her social life. There should *be* a social life; it should include peers with whom she can compete in some areas and from whom she gains some social acceptance. The teen years are the beginning of division into social groups, or cliques, and that may actually fit into your teen's social needs. We are back at the question of whether to be in the mainstream world, be with the disabled, or split the difference. Your teen needs a few friends with whom she shares activities and a confidant relationship. The activities should include occasional evening or weekend forays; they should not be restricted to family or school events. In order to achieve these relationships, your teen might best be exposed to many different people and many different experiences. Some of these should probably be with other disabled persons, whether they are met casually, in school, at camp, or in special recreational or social clubs and programs. The quality of the relationship and the fun they have is the most important thing, and it is unfortunate when either parent or child puts restrictions on the kind of person with whom she may associate, especially when disabled people are excluded. Some of the more unsatisfactory solutions are socializing only with parents and other adults, attending only occasional mainstream functions without establishing close relationships, or not socializing at all.

It sometimes takes persistence and a great deal of effort on the part of child and parent to establish and maintain social relationships. Appropriate groups must be found, whether it be the camp, the receptive Boy Scout or Girl Scout troop, the social club, or the park recreation program. Friendships must be cultivated, and if they are to be cultivated they need a place to happen, whether it be a movie, pizza palace, church youth house, park, or someone's home. It should be a place where teens can enjoy reasonable privacy and the opportunity to make at least a minor rumpus. Teens in a group are loud. Teens also need some limits within which they can operate independently, making their own decisions about when and where to go. While that can be difficult to achieve, especially if they require special transportation, it is worth the effort to provide as much leeway as possible.

There is no more critical factor in the disabled teenager's social and recreational development than transportation. Parents should make every effort to make transportation as easily and flexibly available as is within their means. Use every resource you can, including sharing with other families, riding with teens who drive, using public transportation such as buses, vans, or taxis. Vote your tax dollars for accessible public transportation!

In addition to needing the capacity to be themselves or to get places easily, teens need flexibility in schedules if they are to test their capacity to make independent decisions and take responsible actions. It is hard for you to learn that their judgment can be trusted if they have no leeway for freedom.

Privacy is obviously important if the teen is to extend her social relationships to dating and, ultimately, to sexual relationships. Imagine trying to form a relationship, male or female, if your mother is always there! Somehow one needs the opportunity to hold hands, steal a kiss, and perhaps do a little groping. Considerable tact and discretion and thoughtfulness are needed, especially where parents are the prime source of transportation or homes the prime location of socializing.

Parents should also try to be tolerant of the telephone network that teens frequently set up and that may be especially important to the teen with mobility limitations. Harry and Lavonne and Mary and Tom and Bill all have severe physical disabilities; all are in wheelchairs. They have a social network that carries them from school to their weekly adolescent group meeting to the Special Olympics to Easter Seal Camp. These events are interlaced with telephone conversations, occasional visits to one another's homes, and other events such as attendance at a dance or rock concert. They keep track of one another, care about one another, and spread personal news faster than the television networks. They are a social unit.

Sexuality is at least as important to teens with disabilities as it is to others. Their bodies grow and they develop secondary sexual characteristics (beards, breasts, and pubic hair) that both please and puzzle them. Their glands secrete and they get impulses. They experiment with themselves, and with others if they get the chance. They need accurate knowledge about sex in general and about their own capacities in particular. If you can provide some or all of the knowledge, that is fine. Be aware that most parents, even with the best intentions, don't seem to succeed in doing this. It is hard to find the right moment and the right words to talk with our teen children about sex. Our experience in talking about sex with groups tells us that many teens are as embarrassed as their parents at first. Although they are often poorly informed, they are usually open to discussion that combines informality with real information giving.

You should see that your teen has the opportunity to learn about sexuality somewhere. Many schools have good sex education programs, and attendance should be encouraged. Sex education may be provided in the context of your church or synagogue. You may want to supplement general sex education with a discussion with health professionals, especially if your teen's disability is related in any way to the ability to function sexually or to be a parent. The possibility of children inheriting the disability may also be an issue. If your teen has been treated by a multidisciplinary team, they may be the persons to whom you wish to turn for information about sexuality. It is usually desirable to set up separate interviews for parents and teens. That way each will be able to ask the questions of greatest interest to him or her and to discuss them according to his or her own level of understanding and interest. This may also allow for frank questions and expression of concerns in a way that might in some families be prevented by embarrassment.

Included in sex education will be birth control methods. Attitudes toward them will, of course, vary according to your religious belief or personal philosophy. At a minimum, your teen should know the facts of procreation, have a general knowledge of the concept of birth control, and know the family's beliefs and attitudes toward birth control methods. Boys and girls should have some knowledge of (and respect for) the responsibility involved in bringing a child into the world. Whether teens are to have birth control methods available, or even encouraged, will remain a matter of individual philosophy.

In the matter of sexuality, Laura's attitude toward her mother was a mixture of amusement and anger. "She's so uptight. She wants me to know things, but she acts like the words *sex* or *breast* or *penis* would burn her tongue. She also acts like talking to me about it would encourage me to do it. I think she thinks I'm having sex all the time. I haven't even had a chance to say no yet. I'm in no hurry, because I'm still too young to get *that* serious about a guy. I wish Mom'd get over it. She doesn't know as much about sex ed as I got in high school. Parents can be a problem!"

Some teens may have special difficulty in handling sexuality. Girls who have limited social opportunities and who are hungry for acceptance may allow themselves to be exploited in order to try to develop or maintain a relationship. Boys with limited social opportunity may believe everything they hear in the locker room and place undue emphasis on sexual conquest as the goal. In making sex the first goal in each instance, they may fail to develop the ordinary social skills and relationships that are a necessary prelude to a sexual relationship and may thus retard their social development.

*   *   *

All the events in your teen's life—learning self-help and responsibility as well as functioning in the family, school, and society—feed into his self-concept, and this self-concept is the basis on which he will plan his future. How well he knows himself will determine the appropriateness of his plans. Whether he has discovered his true strengths, as well as his limitations, will determine the regard and respect that he has for himself. All of these underline the importance of discovering those things the teen can do well and giving him accurate feedback.

A sense of competence and commitment may be gained in many of life's activities. In school the teen may enjoy academic fields such as language, math, or science; he may also enjoy artistic areas such as music, art, or drama; it could be sports or it could be social functions such as clubs or student politics. Some teens have their major commitments outside of school, in church youth group, Y, Scouts, or other activities. It is important that your teen find something that he enjoys, that involves commitment and time, and in which he gains some extra knowledge or expertise. It may be recreational or social.

In some instances it is worthwhile to provide special training in recreational skills. This may be something at a high level of skill or complexity, like skiing or bridge, but it might equally well be the painstaking learning of more elementary skills, such as playing checkers, four-square, dominoes, Ping-Pong, rummy, fish, or Parcheesi. Again, it should include the development of some knowledge or expertise. It is these activities, these commitments, these special skills around which self-concept are built and from which life goals and programs are developed.

*   *   *

The life of your teen should include, in addition to
school, recreational, and social functions, some activities that are labeled as work. Central to these are
chores, which have already been discussed. In addition,
where opportunities exist, there should be work that
generates some income for the teen. This might range
from babysitting to garden work to part-time employment in a fast food restaurant or car wash. Some high
schools include work experience as part of the school
program. Whenever teens are employed, care should be
taken to see that they have time for sufficient sleep as
well as for academic, social, and recreational needs. Work
should especially not interfere with school. Given a
proper balance, however, gainful employment can go a
long way to developing the teen's work habits (getting
there on time, accepting supervision, getting the job
done), vocational skills, and vocational interests, not to
mention providing a supplement to his allowance.

Handling money is another part of your teen's development that will be closely tied to his maturity and
future competence. He should have some money that is
clearly his to spend, save, or invest as he sees fit. In
today's world, when one takes into account the demands
of school and the limited work opportunities for teens,
an allowance from parents is virtually a requirement. It
is quite fair that the allowance be expected to cover
recreational and social expenses as well as special items
of clothing. It is not fair to call paying the cost of
necessities such as school lunch or basic clothing an
allowance. The use of the allowance must be at least
partly discretionary. Allowance should also not be tied
too directly to chores, lest the meaning of the chores be
lost. Chores are a part of the basic responsibility assumed
by every member of a household. They should not be

done to earn money. Of course, compensation can be provided for duties beyond the ordinary, such as painting the house or waxing the car. In any event, your teen should have the experience of working for pay, and care should be taken that whenever he is employed at least some of the compensation should be made available to him to use for things that he could not otherwise enjoy.

In addition to the many activities we have discussed, the teen years are a time of thinking and talking about life. Your teen may discover, or for the first time realize the importance of, differences between herself and others. She may become aware of limitations that will not change. She may for the first time realize that she will not grow out of her disability. She may discover that others will not treat her in the same way as her parents have and that, indeed, there *is* unfairness and even cruelty in life. If you have established a pattern of open dialogue with your teen, that will help to some extent. Expect to hear expressions of frustration and anger about limits that are real as well as about barriers encountered and judgments met that are based on necessary and unfair stereotypes. Tolerate letting off steam so long as it is not excessive or destructive.

However, be reminded that this is also the time for beginning independence from parents, a time when it becomes important to have a separate identity. Your teen may accomplish much of her thinking and sharing through "rapping" with peers. She may avail herself of a friendly teacher, school counselor, or youth minister. In some instances it may be helpful to seek professional counseling from a psychologist or social worker who is experienced in working with teens and has knowledge of disability. Many teens find it useful and enjoyable to participate in organized groups for handicapped teens, which may be offered through state crippled children's services or other agencies. Such groups usually involve discussion of mutual problems, development of social skills, and planning for the future. They may also serve as a focus for social activity and social contacts.

6

GOING OUT IN THE WORLD
The Young Adult Years

The time for your grown child to bring it all together is during the last year in public school. Knowledge of where she is, who she is, what she can do and what she can't will be the basis of a plan for her career and her residence. Granted, there may be a way to go in developing further skills, and there may be some unanswered questions. Can I make it through this course of training, in that kind of job, living in that sort of setting? But these are the kinds of questions faced by every young adult, with or without a disability. The goals should be set at a level that is optimistic but achievable. They should be based on experiences in the past of doing for oneself at home, completing courses and training in school, dealing with people at large, and doing what work has been available.

In this section we will review and enumerate those tasks or skills the young adult should now be capable of performing. In describing them, we recognize that some functions will be carried out by ordinary means, in an ordinary amount of time, and at an ordinary level of effectiveness. Other functions may be handled by adapting them (Sue's work was arranged so that it could be done sitting down instead of standing), doing them with help (Stanley had an aide in the morning to assist with dressing), or arranging activities so that certain requirements are eliminated (Ellen found work that could be done at home by telephone so that she did not have to travel to a job site). No one can be expected to do what is physically or mentally impossible for him or her. These skills, then, are those the young adult *ideally* should have attained by this time. It is recognized that some persons may be unable to attain all of them because of physical or mental impairment, and in that sense they are only guidelines or ideal goals. But that is the only sense in which learning the skills is optional. *If the person is physically and mentally capable of doing them, these skills are not optional at all; they are mandatory!*

By the end of the school years the luxury of postponement is running out. For example, the young adult may be planning to do clerical work. She now lives with her family a few miles out in the country, beyond the bus line. She does not drive. "We'll work it out when the time comes" is not enough. All involved (most especially the young adult) should be actively working toward an arrangement which involves: 1) the young adult moving out of the family home to residence in the city; *or* 2) learning to drive with adaptive equipment; *or* 3) identifying a source of transportation (volunteer or car pool) that will be reliably available for a long time; *or* 4) the whole family moving to the city; *or* 5) identifying employment that can be done in the home and that can reasonably be expected to be available; *or* 6) identifying a long-term source of funds (such as from a well-paying job) to pay for a driver or taxi service. The point of this example is that tangible plans and actions are needed for many different aspects of transition and that they cannot be put off until the day the transition is to begin.

By now, the young adult should have mastered all those self-help skills of which he is capable and should know how the others will be accomplished. This involves bathing, dressing, and toileting, including a method for getting to and using toilet facilities in public places. The young adult should know how to shop for clothing, choose the appropriate outfit for each day's activity, and care for his apparel, including its laundering and storage.

He should know how to feed himself or find the help he needs. This will include eating in public places like cafeterias and making appropriate choices from the menu. He should know the basics of food preparation, including preparation of simple hot foods (soup, hot drinks). If he is living independently he should have more advanced food preparation skills (stews, casseroles) as well as the ability to shop for groceries, showing some consideration for a balanced diet as well as cost.

The young adult should have the capacity to get about in his community for work, recreation, and social purposes. Learning to drive a car is highly desirable, if feasible. Mastering the public transportation system (bus or train) is the next-best key to independent mobility. If special transportation is necessary, he should be able to make the arrangements (phone calls, etc.) himself. Ideally, the young adult should also be able to use long-distance air or ground transportation services, so that visits to distant friends and relatives or vacation trips are possible. It should be pointed out that there is a real difference between being able to do these things hypothetically and actually doing them. Parents and others will often say, "Oh, Joe could ride the bus if he needed to or make those arrangements by phone if he had to." When it comes time for Joe to do it, it is discovered that many things were overlooked or taken for granted. A great deal can be gained by insisting that young adults get actual practice in such skills, because such practice will prepare them to do them when they need to and because it gives them new abilities and confidence for handling other situations.

The young adult should have the skills needed to develop and maintain social relationships. Among these are the capacity to be interested in someone else and to follow a conversational lead. They should include the basic social skills that make people comfortable, such as *hello, goodbye, please,* and *thank you,* giving eye contact during conversation, and acknowledging communication received. These social skills are also needed to maintain good employment relations. Other required work habits include getting there on time or calling in if delayed; sustaining effort until the job is done; accepting supervision, including constructive criticism; and placing social needs secondary to work activities while on the job. It cannot be assumed that the young adult will somehow have social skills in a job setting that he has not previously had in school or at home. We remember an appointment to provide vocational evaluation and career counseling to Allen, a young man of nineteen, who was mildly retarded in his mental functioning. He was a tall and muscular fellow, the only child of his elderly parents, who accompanied him. As we met in the lobby they introduced him by saying, "We brought him in to see about getting a job." Not ten minutes later, in the initial interview, the same parents were

saying, "Oh, he never goes anywhere without us along."
They saw no discrepancy in those two statements. Allen
did have good job potential. About two years were spent
in providing him with the training and experience in the
prevocational skills (getting to work alone, eating in the
cafeteria, accepting supervision from others) he would
need to hold a job. All these skills were ones that could
have been more comfortably learned in the early teen years.

The young adult should have developed certain patterns of responsibility while growing up, like getting
himself up in the morning and anticipating his needs for
the day, such as transportation or a bag lunch. He should
have the ability to be responsible for himself alone at
home all day, to the point where he can be alone overnight (if this is physically and mentally feasible). He
should know his health needs, anticipate and arrange
treatment, and carry out self-treatment such as exercises, injections, or taking pills. Ultimately he should
begin to realize that mastery of these functions means
true independence in that he can decide how and when,
and even if, they will be carried out. He should begin to
appreciate the inevitable and unavoidable fact that *the
price of dependency is not having control*, and he should
not like that. Concurrently, the parents should begin to
appreciate the fact that the price of having a child who
is independent will be the loss of their ability to control,
and they *should* like that. George Preston, a mental
health professional and writer, once wrote in his book
The Substance of Mental Health: "Children are peculiar
possessions. If you care for children properly, you lose
them." (New York: Holt, 1965, p. 27).

A word should be said here for those who have older
children who haven't attained this independence. You
may be reading this and saying, for whatever reason,

"Well, Tom never achieved this. He can't go out alone. He doesn't care for his room or his clothes. He'd starve if someone didn't fix him a meal. It's too late for him now, he's twenty-seven." Or you may be Tom, thinking the same thing about yourself. The answer is that it's never too late, and the place to start is in the home. There is no substitute. No agency or school is likely to start at the beginning to teach those skills. So begin with the chores, with elementary laundry folding and bed making. Teach sandwich making. Arrange jaunts to the neighbors, to the store down the street, and then on the city bus. Get involved in an activity center or workshop. Break up attitude patterns that are person-specific, such as "He won't let anyone but his mother help with his toileting" or "He won't go anywhere unless his father is with him." It won't be easy and the results won't be perfect (as with a person who doesn't learn to drive until his middle years), but it can be done and there's really no substitute. Get professional consultation. Satisfaction in living, and perhaps even maintaining life itself, will depend upon a minimum capacity to care for self and the ability to live with others in the later years.

During the last year in school the teen should begin to narrow the range of career goals that she will consider and ultimately pursue. Work identity is often, but not always, central to a person's life; some people get their greatest sense of competence and life meaning from being an artist, a master bridge player, a volunteer worker, a pillar of the community club or church, or a sports expert, rather than from their paid job. What is important is that there be some central core of activity and interest that a person enjoys and can do to her own level of satisfaction. If that activity is paid employment, then it may also be the person's source of financial support. If it is not, then the person must solve her problems of subsistence in other ways, such as by holding a job or by having other sources of income.

Most vocational goals will require training beyond that available in the public schools. The goal the person sets for herself, plus her level of ability, will determine whether she should plan for training in a four-year college, community college, vocational or business school, an on-the-job setting, a sheltered workshop, or a work activity center. Many persons have a general idea of their strengths, weaknesses, interests, and goals, but find it difficult to organize that knowledge into a plan. Vocational evaluation and career counseling can be invaluable to these persons, whether or not they have a disability. For some persons with serious unanswered questions about their vocational future, vocationally oriented evaluation is indicated *as they enter* the high school years. For one student the question may be whether she has the capacity to do four-year college work in the future and therefore should take college preparatory courses throughout the high school years. For another student the question may be whether she will have the capacity to complete the basic requirements for a high school diploma or whether she would do better to concentrate on work experience, vocational, and survival skills. Still other students may have no problem choosing their high school curriculum but may require help during the last years of school to determine their direction after high school.

Some evaluation and counseling is available through public school programs, although many schools do not provide the individualized approach that is needed when the person has a serious impairment of hearing, vision, or physical dexterity. In some states evaluation and counseling is offered through the state crippled children's service. Many colleges and community colleges operate counseling centers that are available to the public. Career counseling services may also be obtained from private practicing psychologists or vocational counselors. It is important that those providing the service be experienced not only in vocational evaluation and counseling but in working with persons with disability.

It is important to know that such counseling is provided for persons with disabilities by the Vocational Rehabilitation Division (VRD), a state agency with which you should be familiar. Every state has a vocational rehabilitation division, service, or agency. Its mission is to help persons with disability become employable. Through either its own staff or by referral to professionals in the community, it provides evaluation, counseling, treatment services required to become employable, training, and placement assistance. VRD may be your primary source of vocational evaluation, *if the agency is willing to provide this service early enough to meet your particular need.* In some states VRD will provide vocational evaluation early enough to help in high school planning (at age fifteen or sixteen) but in other states VRD will not provide evaluation until the applicant is approaching the end of her public school training. Most states serve separately those persons who are legally blind, through an agency called the Commission for the Blind. These agencies are available to all residents with disability. (The services of VRD are further described in Chapter Thirteen.)

A final word about training and employment: Some persons with disability may need transitional experiences in order to prepare themselves for the training or the job they want. For example, it may be worthwhile to begin college training in a community college, with less intense academic competition, until study habits are refined and new social skills are developed outside the high school setting. Other persons may need to develop work skills and habits in a sheltered workshop before moving on to another training setting or an entry-level job.

Where to live in the future is the major question that parallels or follows the question of what kind of work you will do. Even though the young person may live with the family for several years after high school, planning should be underway so that the necessary skills may be learned and arrangements made that will permit eventual transition from the parental home. For some persons, moving away from family (to a group home, for example) may be necessary to help them develop the social skills needed for independence and vocational competence.

There is a spectrum of options: staying at home, living in an adult foster home, living in a group home, living in a satellite apartment, living independently. Often a plan will involve transition from one to another. The young adult may move into a group home where he will increase his housekeeping skills, learn to live with persons his age, develop friendships and patterns of social and recreational activity, and learn to get about the community. He may then want to move into a satellite apartment, where he will have one or two roommates and where remote supervision is provided. Eventually he may want to rent his own accommodations, which may be shared with a roommate or spouse.

In some instances, families have even looked on living in a group home as an interim experience like going off to school. After a few years of caring for his own needs, dealing with peers, and enjoying social and recreational activities in the group setting, the young adult may plan to move back home. Hopefully he will bring with him a sense of independence and a set of relationships that he will maintain. He may also opt not to return to the family setting. All of these options are discussed further in Chapter Fourteen.

The matter of separation from family in such living arrangements is a matter for some consideration. It is necessary that the person be allowed to make the transition and that others do not accompany him, do it for him, or encourage him to come home again at the first bit of difficulty or discomfort. There will be some difficulty and discomfort: coping with new people, developing new skills and new tastes, periods of frustration and loneliness. The person must know that he is not abandoned but also that others expect him to make it on his own and have confidence he can do it. Sufficient time and space must be allowed for that to happen. *After the transition has been made* (which may require two to six months), there can be opportunity to go home for visits and to share social activities. The eventual goal should be to have a pattern of relationship and activity such as would be expected with other members of the family who are out on their own.

We have discussed two major transitions: vocation and residence, working and living. In helping the young adult plan and carry these out, it is usually wise to set up one major venture at a time. It may be overwhelming, for example, to move into a group home and start a new job or training program at the same time. It may be useful to postpone the move until the job or training program has been underway for several months, or vice versa, to move into the new setting a few months before training or work begins.

Making the transition to independent living is not easy for anyone, with or without disability. Many of us remember our own experience in moving out on our own. For some persons with extensive or severe areas of disability it can be painfully difficult. Issues of dependence must be met: psychological dependence on parents or others and physical dependence for vital functions. It is a time for exploring possibilities. It may be necessary to create options, such as arranging an independent living situation for just a limited period of time. Trial and error is often needed to find the right set of circumstances that will work. It is a time when there may well be some failures and when failure should be seen as a prelude to trying again or trying something new, rather than as a reason for retreat. Alice is thirty-two years old, with severe cerebral palsy. She has just moved into her own apartment ("I can't stand living with anyone else"). Several times in the past she has returned to live briefly with her parents. She has a good clerical job but thinks about getting something more exciting. She has driven adapted vehicles but never owned her own. She is working on getting a van. She cheerfully says, "I'm still learning how to do it. I don't know if I'll ever feel like I've arrived." Everyone involved—parent and, especially, young adult—can expect periods of frustration and anger and depression to be mixed in with the good feelings of accomplishment. It is a time to provide each other with the maximum of tolerance, flexibility, and mutual support.

*   *   *

Marriage is a state with which we all need to reckon in one way or another as we enter adulthood. Our attitude toward it, while not often put into words, is somewhat like our attitude toward a career: Do we want it? What can we aspire to? Will we be competent at it? Will *anyone* want us? Feedback to the disabled person about marriage should be much like that regarding any other aspiration, leaving possibilities open and pointing the way to the first steps, such as having a social life, making friends, dating, financing the date, and so on. No unrealistic promises or predictions, but lots of support and as much optimism as can be justified.

Adolescents and young adults, like the rest of us, are sexual beings—probably more so. All adolescents and young adults, disabled or not, will have a sexual life of some kind, solitary or social. They are entitled to that, and to feel comfortable with it. Most disabled persons are able to have sexual relationships, and they should be helped to pursue them in an informed, dignified, and responsible way. This means information about sexuality, help in learning the skills to develop social relationships that can become sexual ones, mobility, privacy, appropriate dress, and the financial means for dating activity. Many, if not all, persons with disability can consider marriage as an option for their future. First and foremost is the ability to form and maintain the relationship with their prospective spouse. Then a workable plan for living together needs to be formulated. There are a variety of possible arrangements: total independence in every way, including financial; living with federal or state subsidies such as Supplemental Security Income (SSI); or living in a setting with remote supervision, consultation, and assistance as needed, such as may be available in a satellite apartment. The major criterion is that the arrangement be one that can be sustained over a period of time.

The matter of becoming a parent should be considered at the time that marriage is contemplated but should be seen as additional, an extension of marriage. Not everyone who is capable of maintaining a satisfactory marriage relationship or of bearing a child is capable of meeting the responsibility inherent in parenting a child, including nurturing, teaching, modeling for it, meeting its emerging needs, and developing the child to a level of adult maturity and competence. Marriage should not take place until the issue of parenting has been settled, either by determining that it can be carried out successfully or by appropriate birth control methods. Issues of sex and marriage are discussed further in Chapter Twelve.

Independence and pride have been our themes. Our intent in this section is to suggest that your child, now grown to a young adult, should have a sphere of activity of her own. This should involve vocational activity at the highest level at which she can function with a feeling of competence and success, whether it be in competitive employment or a sheltered work setting. It should include activities she looks forward to with enthusiasm, whether they be vocational, recreational, or social. It should include some concern for helping others. While some of her activities may be carried out with family, for the most part they should be with others: friends, co-workers, roommates, spouse.

Not the least of the reasons for emphasizing the ultimate *independence* of activities is emotional well-being and life satisfaction for you, the parents. You

deserve a life of your own. You *need* a life of your own if
you are to be a model for your adult daughters and sons
and if you are to be available to them as a whole and
interesting person who can become friend and peer as
well as parent. Devoting your life to a sphere of activity
that involves only you and your child will be a disser-
vice to both. Move out and live. Enjoy the parade!

SOURCES OF ADDITIONAL INFORMATION

Coombs, J. *Living with the Disabled: You Can Help.*
New York: Sterling Publishing Co., 1984.
A family guide directed primarily to the newly
disabled adolescent and adult. Deals with hospitals,
convalescence, and rehabilitation. Has a useful listing of associations for various disabilities and for
specific types of services.
The Exceptional Parent. 605 Commonwealth Avenue,
Boston, MA 02215.
Magazine published eight times a year. Presents a
wide range of information about law, technology,
programs, and interesting activities of persons with
disability.
Fassler, J. B. *Helping Children Cope.* New York: The
Free Press, 1978.
This book is a guide to children's literature on
topics of stress-producing situations such as hospitalization and illness, death and separation. It suggests books and stories that can be read to and with

children that might assist them in dealing with stressful events.

Hale, G., ed. *The Source Book for the Disabled: An Illustrated Guide to Easier More Independent Living for Physically Disabled People, Their Families and Friends.* New York: Bantam, 1981.

A comprehensive how-to book with sections on daily living skills, leisure and recreation, sexuality, and other relevant topics. Includes an extensive list of resource organizations and publications.

Lindemann, J.E., ed. *Psychological and Behavioral Aspects of Physical Disability: A Manual for Practitioners.* New York: Plenum, 1981.

Discusses the psychological problems associated with thirteen chronic disabling conditions, including cerebral palsy, spina bifida, progressive muscle disorders, sensory impairments, and others. Also contains brief descriptions of the etiology, diagnosis, and treatment of each disability. Addressed primarily to health-care professionals.

Lindemann, J.E., and S.J. Lindemann. "A Typology of Childhood Disorders and Related Support Services," *Childhood Disability and Family Systems*, ed. M. Ferrari and M.B. Sussman. New York: The Haworth Press, 1987.

Contains a useful checklist and description of the support services that may be required by disabled children in six categories: family, medical, financial, educational, psychosocial, and vocational.

Miezio, P.M. *Parenting Children with Disabilities: A Professional Source for Physicians and Guide for Parents.* New York: Dekker, 1983.

Written for both professionals and parents. Contains

discussion of psychological and social problems as well as medical needs.

News Digest: Information from the National Information Center for Handicapped Children and Youth. Free subscriptions. Write: NICHCY, Box 1493, Washington, D. C. 20013.

Short articles about various aspects of disability. Includes many references for their sources of information.

Roy, R. *Move Over, Wheelchairs Coming Through!* New York: Clarion Books, 1985.

Seven young people in wheelchairs talk about their lives. The book focuses how they get around, what they do for recreation, what they do in school, what problems they have, and how they feel about it all.

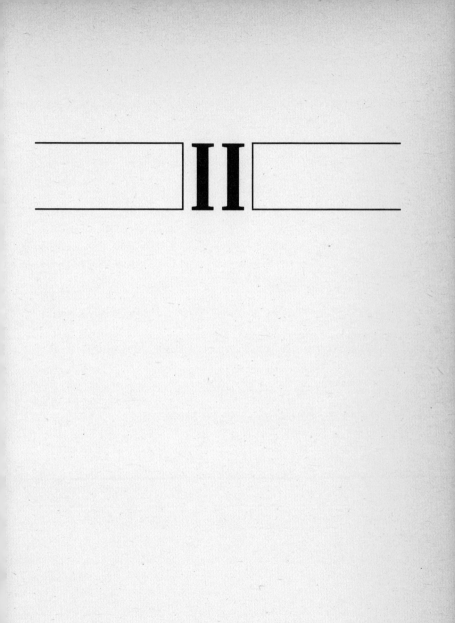

II

7

Training the Child

A child who knows no limits on his behavior is a child who will have difficulty with his peers. In Part I of this book you have learned that children with disabilities are as much in need of expectations, limits, and discipline as are others. This point is emphasized because parents and others find it so easy to overlook unacceptable behavior in a child with disability, to the child's detriment. It can be difficult to make demands on a child who must exert unusual effort simply to manage everyday accomplishments like getting dressed. We recall a mother with tears in her eyes saying, "I know I shouldn't let Fred get away with those things, but I remember how much his uncle [who also had hemophilia] had to suffer when he grew up, and I can't deprive him of anything!" She overlooked the fact that her son was growing up with treatment that minimized the suffering. We know Fred now as a young adult who is having difficulty learning to cope. Sympathy is a powerful emotion and hard to resist. If we allow it to control us so that we do not set limits and appropriate expectations, it is the child who loses in the end.

This chapter will briefly state some principles and practical suggestions for training children in behavior that is independent and self-responsible—and disciplined. For a detailed presentation of principles and techniques of child training, you can refer to the resource books on training listed at the end of this chapter. Should you encounter persistent difficulty in child training and decide that you require extra assistance, you should seek a parent training course offered through a responsible community agency or the services of a licensed psychologist who specializes in working with children and families.

The emphasis here is on training from the start for independent and responsible behavior, with correction or discipline reserved only for the occasional persistent problem. Independence and self-responsibility, of course, are just words, words that describe a large number of small skills and habits built up over a long period of time. Teaching the young child to extend his arm for his sweater (and praising him for it) is the beginning of teaching him to put on the sweater himself. Teaching the schoolchild that the hour after dinner is homework time, to be spent at the study desk or table, is the beginning of teaching him the responsibility for planning homework and getting assignments finished on time, which later becomes an important work characteristic. This is a good news/bad news situation. The good news is that intangible things like independence and responsibility can be taught, and the opportunities to do so are present every day. The bad news is that it takes time—developing patterns of appropriate behavior is done in small increments and is not a matter of one day (at age fifteen, let's say) deciding to change one's attitude.

How does this training get done? We would like to emphasize two major aspects of child training: 1) the quality of your relationship and communication with the child, and 2) the technique of catching him doing something right and praising him for it, an important part of the method of child training, that is commonly known as behavior modification.

Good communication is essential to a good relationship with your child. One way to promote this is to talk about what you're doing and why you're doing it, even with the very young child. "We're putting on your jacket so you'll be warm outside." "Breakfast time! Your tummy will feel good and you'll have lots of energy." Your talk may convey your personal reasons for a request, such as "I can't enjoy my book with that racket in my ear, so please do it in the other room." These are the preferable alternative formulations to "Hold still while I put on your jacket!" "Eat!" and "Stop that racket!" Explaining requests or commands not only helps the child understand but also helps you to be sure that what you are asking or doing is not unreasonable. Obviously one does not carry on this type of chatter all the time, but enough so that the child attaches language to action. Some requests or commands may ask for personal privilege, such as "I know I said I'd do it now, but I'm sorry I can't. I'm just too exhausted. I know you're disappointed, and I promise to do it later." Notice that you recognize the child's feelings and accept them. Of course, children should also be granted personal privileges at times. A word of caution: children who have developed good verbal skills early sometimes wield verbal power over parents before the children have the maturity to make appropriate decisions. They become skilled at argument without a sense of responsibility to go with it. Avoid verbal battles over decisions that are a parent's responsibility. In the long run the child will appreciate the fact that you are in charge.

Listening to the child is equally important to the communication. A great deal of fussing and resistance is often based on the very real reason that young children are unable to communicate because they don't have the words. Parents frequently become skilled at listening so that they can distinguish the "wet cry" from the "pain cry" or the "just vocalizing cry." Observing what infants smile or laugh at can give clues to what things they are paying attention to and what they are getting ready to understand.

Some children are difficult to "read" or to understand. This can be especially true in children whose ability to reason or understand is limited or whose language and speech ability is impaired. It may not only be difficult to understand those children but also difficult to know what they are ready to learn. Parents may assume that a child is ready to learn names, colors, or shapes and may spend a great deal of time repeating, demanding, and being exasperated about things that the child cannot yet comprehend. They may even mistake this inability for obstinance. Casey is a slow-learning child whose progress was frustrating to his parents. They felt he should know his colors and were trying to teach him the printed words that went with the colored blocks. Occasionally he made a correct match, but his errors were interpreted as "He knows how—he just doesn't want to do it now!" It was suggested that the parents' expectations be adjusted to a task that Casey could do at the moment, consistently match blocks of the same color. This was generalized to other objects by having a color of the week in which a game was made of finding red, blue, or green objects in the environment and learning to discriminate and generalize. As Casey became consistent in his ability to match and identify colors, he started receiving much-needed praise and appropriate self-satisfaction rather than thinly veiled disapproval. Parents with a child who is "difficult," especially regarding paying attention, learning, and applying information, are urged to obtain consultation from a professional, such as a psychologist, who can provide help in interpreting behavior and readiness.

Establishing good communication in the early stages can go a long way to reducing problems in the future, so our emphasis is on letting the child know what is going on and understanding his reaction. Note however that understanding the child does not mean that the parent is not the final decision maker, especially when the parent possesses knowledge or judgment that the child does not have and that is necessary to the decision to be made.

Your good relationship and communication with the child are the necessary backdrop for the use of your major tool in child training, the reinforcement of desirable and appropriate behavior.

Your child "behaves" all the time, doing things that express his feelings and impulses and that he expects will get him those things that he wants or needs. It is your job as parent to help him develop behavior that works, and will be effective in expressing himself and getting things in an appropriate way, without unnecessary disruption, destruction, or waste of energy. If he is able to develop that appropriate behavior, the undesirable or ineffective behavior will drop away. You guide and develop his behavior by seeing that his appropriate attempts are rewarded (reinforced)—by being successful, bringing about a pleasant experience (food, warmth, praise), or ending an unpleasant one (cold, pain). You catch him doing something right and reward him for it. You reward his first attempts even if they are not totally effective so they will be repeated and can be built upon in the future. Learning behavior so that it becomes habitual is a slow process. It is also irregular and un- even; backsliding is to be expected, and you must expect that repetition will be necessary.

Rewards (or reinforcements) can be many things. They can be getting what you want, like a toy that was out of reach; they can be a pleasant sensation, like the taste of something sweet; they can be a hug, a smile, or words of approval. As we grow older the appropriate rewards become more social and abstract, including smiles, words of approval, grades in school, money, titles, and public recognition.

The principle with which we are working is that everyone, including your child, learns to use behavior that works. Thus, if the child pees on the rug or throws his banana pudding and discovers that everyone laughs and thinks it is cute, he will do it again. Similarly, if by throwing a tantrum he is able to avoid going to bed, he will do that again. On the other hand, if he gets praise and a gold star for using the toilet, or Mom notices when he is neat and hugs him for it, or Dad reads him a short story after he is in his PJ's and in bed, then he will do those things again.

Sometimes you can set up the situation so that the desired behavior is likely to occur. For example, if the child is learning to walk with braces and needs practice, you may set an attractive toy at a reasonable distance and praise the child for walking to it. Sometimes you may want to keep track of desired behavior (brushing teeth, completing homework) or undesired behavior (teas- ing little brother, coming in late, doing wheelies in the street). Such records are best kept in a public place, such as on a chart that hangs on the bathroom or refrigerator door. Reaching a certain level of desired behavior or minimizing undesired behavior may then be rewarded at the end of the day, week, or month as appropriate. Rewards may be a small gift, a privilege such as staying up for the late show, money, or points toward a larger reward such as a trip to a rock concert. In general, the more promptly the child is rewarded (even if it is only with points or a star), the more likely he is to learn that behavior.

Situations that bring out undesirable behavior are best seen by parents as problems to be solved rather than as issues to be avoided. To say "I'm never going to take him to a supermarket (restaurant, ball game, theater) again!" is an understandable response by the exasperated parent. Unfortunately, if carried out it will prevent the child from having guided opportunities to learn. Your time would be well invested in figuring out how to introduce the child to these settings gradually (short trip to the store, restaurant for a Coke only, children's theater) and look for opportunities to schedule such experiences at a time when you are not hurried and the child is in a positive mood.

The way in which behavior is weakened, unlearned, or eliminated is by *not* rewarding or reinforcing it. Frequently, rewarding the positive and ignoring the negative will be enough. Sometimes undesirable behavior is given negative reinforcement by withholding a privilege, such as permission to watch TV, have a favorite toy, or go out on a weekend night. Sometimes the non-rewarding is given special emphasis by putting a child in what is called *Time Out*. *Time Out* is a condition in which the child is denied the ordinary rewards of being with people

or in an interesting setting. *"Time Out"* means placing
the child in an uninteresting place, such as a small room
with just a chair or the bathroom (with medications,
radio, and anything else of interest removed). He is placed
there for a specified, short (two-to-three-minute) period
of time, usually as a consequence of undesired behavior
such as a tantrum or flagrant noncompliance. After the
specified interval he may return to the normal setting
and remain there, providing the undesirable behavior is
no longer displayed. The whole procedure should be
carried out in a matter-of-fact way, without anger. It is
important that the *"Time Out"* place not be dark,
frightening, or in any way dangerous. It is not punish-
ment, it is simply a place where the child does not
experience the ordinary rewards of dealing with people
or carrying on his daily activities.

The development of routines is helpful in training,
especially with young children who take well to meals,
baths, and playtime, being on a schedule they can learn.
This also includes routines, so that coming in the
door includes hanging up your coat and going to bed
includes picking up the toys. Consistency in training
children is also important in that the child should not
be allowed to do something one day and forbidden the
next, or permitted by one parent to do an activity which
is forbidden by the other. He should also not be given
conflicting demands ("Go to bed!" followed by "Clean
your room!" for example) so that it is impossible to
comply successfully with all of them.

It is important to realize that rewarding desirable
behavior and not rewarding undesirable behavior is a
teaching method for you, the parent, and a necessary
learning experience for the child. It is the way we *all*
learn what is effective in achieving our needs and in

getting along with others. Children are not born with a built-in sense of right or wrong, good or bad; they learn it. So you are not only teaching your child what is effective; you are teaching him values. The major point is that you are not "bribing" him to do what is right but *teaching* him to do what is right, based on your values as a parent.

The principle of rewarding desired behavior is especially useful for developing appropriate everyday behavior. It may also be used to solve problems such as noncompliance, temper tantrums, bedwetting, and a host of others. For such applications, please see the books on training listed at the end of this chapter or turn to appropriate sources of professional help such as mentioned previously.

SOURCES OF ADDITIONAL INFORMATION

Becker, W.C. *Parents Are Teachers: A Child Management Program*. Champaign, IL: Research Press, 1971. Teaches the basics of behavior modification and how it can be used in child training. Discusses applications in common problem situations.

Patterson, G.A. *Living with Children: New Methods for Parents and Teachers*, revised ed. Champaign, IL: Research Press, 1980. An introduction to child training through behavior modification methods. Includes how-to instructions for dealing with common parental concerns such as temper tantrums, noncompliance, and toilet training. Also describes applications to more severe difficulties of problem children.

8

Adaptive Behavior Skills

Adaptive behavior skills are the building blocks of personal independence. They include the skills that are used for eating, dressing, personal hygiene, mobility, communication, socialization, and self-responsibility. To the extent that we develop these skills to an adult level we are independent of others and have feelings of confidence and self-reliance. They may be achieved completely. They may be achieved through adaptive equipment or methods. They may be achieved with partial or total assistance from other persons, such as a parent or attendant. Most of them are learned in the home. Few disabilities affect all areas of adaptive behavior, and most people with disability are able to function to some extent in each of the areas. The range of life activities in which your child can participate will depend upon the development of a practical method for functioning in each of the skill areas. Like all skills, each activity begins at a simple level and progresses to the more complex. The kinds of skills are essentially the same for all persons, with or without disability.

Eating skills begin when you feed the child and she learns to find the nipple or hold the bottle. They progress to eating at the table and mastering the use of each of the utensils—spoon, fork, and knife for both spreading and cutting. They include not only holding the cup but getting her own glass of water and pouring the milk. Your child should learn food preparation, beginning with getting food from the refrigerator, making sandwiches, and then heating soup or hot drinks. Clearing the table and washing and drying dishes is part of the process. By the teen years your child should master, within her ability, all of those skills she would need to live independently in an apartment: cooking meats, vegetables, and casseroles; planning a balanced diet; and shopping with an eye to values. Some people develop these skills to a point where they are a social asset, such as when they learn gourmet cookery and use it for entertaining. In tandem with her home eating skills, your child should learn to eat in a restaurant, choose from a menu, and manage a cafeteria line by doing it herself or asking for help if needed.

Dressing skills begin when the baby learns to accept diapering without protest and later to extend her feet for shoes. Helping to undress comes first, then dressing, including putting on pants, managing buttons and zippers, and tying shoes. This progresses to dressing independently, including choice of clothing appropriate to the occasion and the weather. Parallel with dressing is the care of clothing, including folding and putting away, then use of the washer and dryer, with selection of the appropriate amount of detergent. Dressing includes purchase of clothing, beginning with simple articles and eventually to all clothing, including choices that take into account quality, style, and value.

Personal hygiene skills begin when the baby cries to have its diaper changed. It progresses to toilet training and learning to wash and dry hands and face. It involves bathing, including care for hair and nails. In girls it includes self-care during menstruation. It extends to the avoidance of contaminated substances and of persons with contagious illnesses. It also includes self-medication for minor pains and illness, skin care to prevent decubiti (skin sores) in those who are paralyzed and/or make regular use of a wheelchair, precautions to prevent kidney infections, routine self-treatment for chronic illnesses such as diabetes or hemophilia, and the capacity to find medical care as needed.

Mobility begins when the baby rolls over, then crawls and walks. She may need to learn to master and care for a walker or wheelchair, or to use braces or crutches. Mobility begins in her room, then about the house, the yard, the neighborhood, and the community. It includes getting into cars, riding the school bus, and finally using public transportation such as the city bus system, special vans, or taxis. Eventually it means distant travel by bus, plane, or train. If at all possible, it should include learning to drive a car—that ultimate symbol of personal freedom in American society.

Communication begins when you exchange coos, squeaks, and smiles with the baby. It progresses when you learn to identify different cries and the baby learns to use them to get a desired result. It is always a two-way process, being expressed and received by the baby and others. It is important to stimulate her nonverbally by smiles and caresses and verbally by naming things and talking about what you're doing. As she develops the capacity to make sounds and words, expect her to name things, too. She will learn to name simple objects, people, colors, and forms. Single words develop into simple sentences, and simple sounds develop into complex pronunciations. Don't worry if the pronunciations aren't exact at first; encourage the child to keep on speaking. Communication progresses to writing, beginning with formless scrawls, and on to block and cursive productions. Be sure your child has access to paper, crayons, and pencils. Communication, as we have said, is a two-way process. It involves both the expression and the comprehension of thoughts. In addition to learning how to comprehend speech, the child will go on to the level of her ability to learn to read and then to express her thoughts in writing. Using a telephone is another part of communication, beginning with talking on it, then answering it, then placing a call.

Socialization begins when the baby smiles in response to your smile, when she reaches for the toy that is offered, and (shudder) when she throws it down to have it picked up for her. It progresses to the recognition of individuals and then to selective responses to people—whether parents, friends, or strangers. It includes playing alongside peers, then playing with them, then participating in structured games with rules. It extends to group participation, as in the classroom. It includes the capacity to choose the right clothing for the situation, such as jeans for labor work, shorts for a picnic, and shirt and tie or dress for the office. It involves complicated patterns of behavior such as those involved in dating, which includes establishing contact, making small talk, setting up the date, choice of appropriate activity (movie, sports event), and on to the complicated understandings that comprise friendship. It includes appreciation of the need to be honest and reliable with others in order to maintain relationships. Social skills must ultimately be developed in relation to peers, as the experience of the child in dealing with adults and parents is not sufficient as preparation for peer relationships. She needs contact with peers outside the family setting.

Self-responsibility begins when the child is left in the room by herself. It extends to the freedom of the house, the yard, the neighborhood, and the community. It develops in time, from a few minutes unattended to a few hours, to home alone all day, and then to overnight. The beginning of the development of self-responsibility is in leaving the child with responsible persons other than parents, continuing on to attendance at school, to visits away from home for a day, then overnight with relatives, then friends and others. It is developed by attendance at camp and at other functions without parental supervision. It includes coming and going, first with permission, then with a simple statement of destination, then freely within certain hours, and finally completely on one's own schedule. It eventually includes responsibility for money, for living arrangements, for entering into contracts, and finally for the care of others.

Virtually all elements of adaptive behavior are learned slowly, in small increments. Most of the learning begins in the home, and some of it can be effectively accomplished only in the home. The twenty years you spend in the parent-child relationship with your son or daughter represent training time, and your home the training ground. It is a time for sharing—of effort and fun, frustration and accomplishment.

It is useful to think of the small actions that make up adaptive behavior skills as habits that become more or less automatic parts of our functioning. We don't *think* about putting on our clothes or washing our hands because we have done it so many times that each part of the process is done without thinking. This repetition is one of the elements of learning, and it is readily applied to teaching your child just about anything. The more times she puts her socks on, the easier it will become. The more times she feeds herself, the more automatic the motions become.

The first thing you must do in teaching your child a skill is to assure yourself that she has the physical and mental capacity to do it. Does Carla have the grip and the strength to get a grasp on a sock and pull it up? Does she have the reasoning ability to handle a job that requires judgments, such as whether something is too big, too small, too hot, or too cold? Can she see as well as necessary to do the task?

Second, you begin teaching by breaking the task into simple elements. The whole act of putting on your socks may be broken into parts so that Carla can learn in easy stages. At first let her feel success by your pulling the sock up over the heel, letting her complete the process you have set up. Next you may put the sock over the toe and she will complete the process from there. Finally she will do it all herself. Training for travel to school or a job may require mastery of parts before the whole can be accomplished successfully. You may walk all the way to school with your child, then only partway, and finally just give her a kiss at the door.

Motivation is important to learning. Even if your child wants (is motivated) to learn a skill, it is important that she know she is doing it correctly and that she be rewarded (reinforced) for doing it. You need to find out how to reward an action and build that into the routine. For many children verbal praise, obvious at first, is all that is needed to encourage them to go through the steps of learning a habit. The amount of praise for a tiny step (pulling up the sock) can be later used for the whole procedure and can be gradually faded out to be used later only occasionally to reinforce the habit ("I'm so pleased with the way you put your socks on without being told!").

After a child has learned to do a task, there may be times when she would rather *not* do it. If you are sure that she has mastered it and that it has been presented positively, with enough time for completion, then it may be time to introduce natural consequences for not doing it. "I know it's easier to wait until I dress you, but I'm not going to do it, even if you are late." "I'm sorry you spent your time playing with your food instead of eating. We're all finished now." Again, avoid being drawn into verbal battles—just state your position and go about your business. Children usually learn that performing simple routines they can handle is preferable to the consequences of not performing them, such as missing a bus or having no more food until the next meal.

Each of the areas of adaptive behavior has been presented here as a continuum, from the simplest to the highest levels. Relatively few persons, disabled or not, accomplish the top level of skill in every area of adaptive behavior. The world has plenty of poor communicators, bad cooks, smelly people, and sloppy eaters. Your child may have a deficit in ability to see or hear, in ability to walk, in hand dexterity or strength, in speech, or in ability to comprehend and make judgments. As a result, it may take a long time to develop skills in some areas. Adaptive equipment or unusual methods may be needed or assistance required. *Your job is to see that limitations in adaptive behavior that persist are not because expectations were not set, not because methods were not tried, not because it wasn't worth taking the time and trouble, and most especially not because you decided (without trying) that it would be just too hard.*

There are times when expediency will get priority, when things must be done by a deadline. But do not allow this to become a chronic behavior; don't fall into the habit of thinking, "It's easier for me to dress her for school than to wait for her to do it." Having your child complete the whole job of dressing for school may mean getting up an hour early for several months, but will be worth it in the end, and the amount of extra time will decrease as proficiency (and the realization that no one is going to do it for her) increases. Similarly, having the awkward child clear the table may mean an occasional broken dish but will also be worth it. (Using plastic or other unbreakable dishes will help. We know a cerebral palsied person who did not learn to set or clear the table until she was an adult because her family refused to give up the use of their china placeware for breakfast or lunch.)

A lot of help is available. There are many books that describe adaptive equipment and adaptive methods. A number of them are listed at the end of this chapter. Occupational therapists are the single best outside source of help and information, followed by physical therapists., pediatricians, psychologists, social workers, speech and language pathologists, and special educators. The single best sources of new ideas, however, are you and your child as well as other parents and children who have similar problems. Over the years we have seen amazing examples of ingenuity on the part of children and parents in working out specific problems. When you realize that you have a persistent difficulty, set up a problem-solving effort. Consult the books, consult the experts, and then have a brainstorming session in the family. Select a strategy and then approach it with trial and error. Allow for mistakes and allow for time. The approaches are many. Velcro as a fastener can perform miracles; elasticized pants and bras that fasten in the front eliminate problems; there are all kinds of adapted eating utensils; boards may be used as a bridge for transferring from wheelchair to toilet; lights that flash can be substituted for things that ring (like doorbells or telephones), and vice versa; and voice-writers and language boards can be great communicators. Think hard about alternative ways of doing things, and be sure to have the family do-it-yourselfers involved in the process. Your job at the end is to see that your child is doing everything of which she is capable. The result will be greater social acceptance from others, more self-confidence for the child, and a justifiably proud (if tired) parent.

In Appendix A you will find a copy of the Portland Tracking System for Adult Living. It can be removed for use, and you may make copies if you need more. It is a listing of those skills that are generally required for independent living as an adult. It can be used as progress sheet, with markings for those skills that have been acquired, those that need attention and further development, those whose attainment is uncertain (may or may not be achievable), and those that are not applicable, either because your child will not be able to achieve them or because they are not necessary. The development of these skills will begin early in life. We suggest that, beginning with the teen years, the list be used for a regular review every six months to provide a record of what has been accomplished and a basis for setting goals for the next six months.

SOURCES OF ADDITIONAL INFORMATION

Blumenfeld, J., et al. *Help Them Grow! A Pictorial Handbook for Parents of Handicapped Children.* Nashville: Abingdon Press, 1971.
Illustrated suggestions for teaching family-living skills, self-help skills, and social skills.

Enrichment Project for Handicapped Infants. *Hawaii Early Learning Profile (HELP): Activity Guide.* Palo Alto, CA: VORT Corporation: P. O. Box 11132. 1979.
Developmental guidelines for children up to three years of age, with suggestions for activities and teaching methods appropriate for handicapped children.

Hale, G., ed. *The Source Book for the Disabled: An Illustrated Guide to Easier More Independent Living for Physically Disabled People, Their Families and Friends.* New York: Bantam, 1981.
This comprehensive how-to book includes a section on useful adaptations and methods for learning self-help skills.

Sargent, J.V. *An Easier Way: Handbook for the Elderly and Handicapped.* New York: Walker & Co., 1981.
Practical, inexpensive suggestions for aids for the physically disabled in areas such as household tasks (cooking, cleaning), personal needs (dressing, grooming, eating), mobility, and so forth. Source references for catalogs and organizations.

9

Education

The education of children is something that takes place every day of their lives. As a parent you will be involved in much of your child's education at home and in school, and must be if he is to use his education effectively. Being involved can be a gratifying experience. This chapter will focus on the part of your child's education that is organized in the form of the school program.

Formal education has traditionally started with first grade or kindergarten, and most special education services begin at these levels. With some disabling conditions, the need for such services might not be evident until the child has begun the process of learning to read and write. In other cases it can be foreseen that children will have difficulty with the school process, and for them enrollment in a preschool is especially important in order to give them the extra help they need to get started. In general, preschool participation is recommended because it provides socialization and an opportunity to learn to function in a class setting. It helps to prepare your child for more formal schooling. In the case of a child with disability it also provides a respite time for the parents. Some district, regional, or state units provide or subsidize preschool programs. Some federally funded programs such as Headstart are required to take a number of handicapped children. Other privately or publicly funded programs may be available in your community.

Early intervention services will be particularly appropriate if your child has a sensory or motor deficit that interferes with communication. This may begin with infant stimulation or parent-child training programs to assist you at beginning levels of communication when severe vision or hearing impairment makes it necessary to develop alternative methods for the child to express himself. If your child is blind, you might be taught to use noisemakers and textured surfaces to provide information and interest to him. You may learn to pair manual signs with objects for the deaf child. These services are often provided by teacher-trainers who come to the home, and they can precede a preschool program.

In preschool your child will learn more about the two-way street of communication. The visually impaired or blind child will learn how to make use of blurred images or of cues he hears or feels in his environment. He also learns the early hand skills that come before the formal learning of Braille as one method of expressing himself. The physically handicapped child whose muscles for producing speech are faulty may learn some basic ways to communicate by making choices and pointing, thus building up a method of expressing himself. The deaf or hearing-impaired child will learn skills that are prerequisites for his method of communicating. This may be either the Total Communication Method or the Oral/Aural Method (see Chapter Sixteen).

For all children the preschool experience can provide not only the specialized training but also practice in dealing with children of their own age and with adults other than their parents. Disabled children need to learn early on that the world isn't going to revolve around them and that they will be required to meet their own needs or seek appropriate help as part of a group of peers.

The subject matter of regular school courses or classes is generally geared to the level of understanding and capability of the average child, with some leeway for children who are slightly above or below the average in their capacity to make use of the material presented. Regular school programs are also primarily geared to presenting material to students who can see, hear, talk, and move about in an ordinary manner. Some schools and individual teachers will be sensitive and motivated to deal with variations in a student's capacity in these areas. As long as your student isn't too far below his age mates in reasoning ability and isn't too limited with sensory or motor deficits, he should be able to take advantage of the mainstream setting with little or no assistance.

If your child has a sensory, motor, or cognitive (reasoning) deficit that interferes with some aspect of learning, specialized services may be needed for him and for his teachers. These are usually described as Special Education Services and should be available according to need. For instance, the child with a mild impairment of his vision may need only the availability of a vision specialist teacher for occasional consultation with the classroom teacher in order to describe the limitations that the student might have and how the teacher might be sensitive to such things as preferential seating, use of clearly printed worksheets, and size of print material. Another child may be severely limited in ability to move, may be in a wheelchair, and may need help with eating, toileting, or medical treatment during the course of the school day. The range of services provided will differ among school districts. Sometimes specialized services are available on a regional basis, with smaller school districts sharing the use of personnel.

At the time your child enters the public school system, decisions should be made regarding his needs in an educational program. (These needs may, of course, change over the years.) You have had consultation and recommendations from those who have been treating him, and the basic requirements of a program may have become evident in the preschool years. It now becomes a matter of getting that information and those recommendations into the hands of the appropriate school personnel.

The need for program planning for children who require special education services was recognized by the action of the federal government in response to parent concern. Public Law 94–142, the Education for All Handicapped Children Act of 1975, requires that "a free and appropriate public education" be provided for all children up through the twenty-first year. The provisions call for evaluation of student needs and construction of appropriate Individual Educational Plans or Programs (IEP's) that are written with the parent, are subject to revision, and include a schedule for monitoring progress. While it is fairly specific about the rights of students to services, the law is differently interpreted, financed, and carried out by the individual states and school districts. There is a due process procedure by which parents can seek further assistance if they are in conflict with their district about their child's program needs.

The law states that the child must be educated in "the least restrictive environment" with regard to classroom placement. This would best be interpreted as the setting that offers the needed services (for example, speech therapy, academic instruction at his functional level, Total Communication, occupational therapy), that offers peer interaction at a level he can take advantage of, and that offers a safe environment. A physically handicapped child who needs a wheelchair for mobility but whose intellectual and academic abilities are on a par with his age peers may need some assistance (ramps, appropriate toilet facilities, physical therapy consultation), but for him the least restrictive educational environment will be the regular or mainstream classroom.

Every student should have the advantage of a setting in which he can receive services or specialized training in relation to his unique abilities or disabilities. For example, placement of a student with markedly limited intellectual abilities in the mainstream might be more restrictive rather than less restrictive in regard to his ability to take advantage of the total school experience. The least restrictive environment for those whose mental ability is limited would be a setting where a lower teacher-to-pupil ratio is present and where content is presented in a format and at a rate they can handle. In general, the more mainstreamed the classroom the better, but not to the point of putting unrealistic expectations on or sidetracking the child. Jackson, a boy with Down's Syndrome, was provided with early parent training services and good preschool services. Through a very structured program and consistency in expectations at home and in school, he was well trained in many developmental skills. At age five, although tests placed him in the moderately retarded range, he was able to perform many of those preschool tasks five-year-olds commonly know, such as naming colors, pointing to body parts, and rote counting. His parents concluded that his greatest need at this point was the presence of good models and interaction with same-age peers, and they enrolled him in a regular kindergarten. By midyear Jackson's friendly temperament had switched to a not-so-cute stubbornness (interpreted by his parents as asssertion of independence), and the attention given to him by the teacher was "What is he doing now?" rather than "Let's think about what he can do next." Having lost the highly structured setting and its low teacher-to-pupil ratio, Jackson became less able to participate effectively and got more negative attention. He was unable to learn new material at a *rate* similar to that of his classmates. His mother had insisted on this placement over the advice of the special education providers who had been serving her child in the preschool years. At the end of the kindergarten year Jackson was reassigned to a smaller classroom with more definite structure and behavioral expectations and where the curriculum could be tailored more to his rate of learning. At the same time, provision was made for many opportunities for interaction with his age peers from "regular" classes in activities such as playtime, music, lunchtime, and field trips. In a setting where he knew what was expected and could keep up with the pace of things, he slowly regained his sunny disposition.

As your child proceeds through the school years you will (and should) become familiar with the array of special education services he may need, whether they be itinerant consultation or a self-contained, highly specialized classroom. You will meet parents of other children who have disabilities. In many places groups have been established to provide assistance with such things as respite services, advocacy, and legislative action. In most states informational materials regarding education for the handicapped, special programs, and the procedures for gaining access to them can be obtained from the state department of education or from designated advocacy agencies. Parents who are well informed and who can provide constructive advocacy for their children are helpful to both their children and others who follow.

Most states have regulations that require that what is known as a handicapping condition be certified in order to qualify for special education services. In addition, there should be a multidisciplinary evaluation aimed at determining your child's program needs. This will be an important step in planning for your child's education. Those doing the evaluation should be experienced and skilled in assessing the abilities of children who are disabled. For instance, a physically disabled child who does not have good use of his arms and hands should be allowed to demonstrate knowledge (tested) in ways that do not require him to use his hands. He should be properly positioned and supported for maximum advantage. The visually impaired or blind child may need to have material presented verbally rather than in printed form. The evaluation process should include information from your treatment team as well as a medical history pertaining to your child's program. At this point, you the parent can supply a great deal of useful information from your personal knowledge of your child's habits and behaviors.

It is very important for you to keep in close contact with the classroom teacher as well as the specialists who might work with your child. Place a teacher conference or classroom visit on the same level of importance as you would a visit to the physician. Your child is spending a *great* deal of time in his school setting, and the more you know about it, the easier it will be for you to participate effectively in the planning process and to make your knowledge of the child a useful part of his school program. It will also put you in a better position should you disagree with elements of the program.

There should be consistency between home and school in expectations for behavior and self-help skills. In our experience, many parents are surprised at what children will do for themselves at school, simply because it is expected as part of the classroom routine. The "He won't do that for *me!*" discovery can lead you to change your expectations and pave the way for increased independence at home. Also, specialists providing service to your child may assist you in learning new techniques of handling your child's needs. Likewise, the teacher may be surprised to learn what the child can do for himself at home and should be expected to do in school. Adapting methods and apparatus to accomplish things like eating, making transfers in and out of wheelchairs, or communicating is an ongoing challenge in which those at home and school personnel can be of great assistance to each other. If your child uses a standard procedure such as manual sign in school, you should take advantage of available sign classes as well as learning the signs your child brings home.

You should also see that communication takes place between the school service providers and the treatment facility you have been using. Again, there should be consistency for the benefit of the student, and if conflict occurs you have an obligation and a right to ask these professionals to share their views and arrive at an acceptable decision about appropriate services.

*   *   *

A variety of specialized classrooms might be available, depending on location. Larger school districts often have a range of settings as well as services. Smaller districts may share services or contract for them as needed.

Some states have residential schools for the deaf and blind as well as the severely mentally handicapped. Residential placement should be approached with caution because of disruption of family relationships, removal from the home community, and in some instances, isolation from contact with a broad spectrum of people. Residential placement may be necessary or useful if it is extremely difficult or dangerous for your child to live in his home or community or if he is in need of highly specialized, twenty-four-hour-per-day training in survival skills in addition to his academic program.

In some areas home instruction services are available to those children whose medical conditions require extended hospitalization or whose conditions, such as limited stamina or unusual susceptibility to infection make classroom attendance difficult or impossible. In considering home teaching, however, great care must be given to balancing the medical needs against the child's need to be in an environment that provides more social stimulation, motivation, and variety in the presentation of information than he will get at home. It is easy to overprotect because of fear or expediency and to make a decision that may not, in the long run, be in the best interests of the child. Better to challenge him somewhat than to isolate him.

Major program decisions will arise at different points in children's school careers. For example, it may become clear early in his schooling that a child will not have the mental ability to master the elements of reading. A common problem occurs when a child appears to be able to read stories that he has actually learned only from constant repetition and is therefore not able to read the same words in a different setting. Teaching or training in survival skills should be given to the child with limited reading ability so that he learns to recognize sign shapes and other more concrete cues to the environment. At a later time such a student may be provided with prevocational and vocational training in which specific practical skills are taught in hands-on situations.

Some children may have difficulty or be slow in understanding the basic principles of reading or arithmetic. Not all children learn these subjects at the same rate. Care should be taken to see that beginning skills are mastered before the child goes on to the next level, where the beginning skills will be taken for granted. Again we see the importance of remaining in contact with the teacher. If your child is having difficulty, ask the teacher to tell you the goals of that subject and how they are taught and tested.

Remember that even though schools may be large and bureaucratic and you may sometimes have difficulty in understanding their ways, they are there for the benefit of you and your child. By and large the school personnel are interested in your child and want to make the system successful. First and foremost, stay in communication with them and help to make school work. Operating in partnership will be more pleasant and more fruitful for your child.

SOURCES OF ADDITIONAL INFORMATION

Cutler, B.C. *Unraveling the Special Education Maze: An Action Guide for Parents.* Champaign, IL: Research Press, 1981.
A guide to rights under P.L. 94–142, special education, the individualized educational program, and advocacy. Clearly written, with examples.

Mitchell, J.S. *See Me More Clearly: Career and Life Planning for Teens with Physical Disabilities.* New York: Harcourt, Brace, Jovanovich, 1980.
Discusses issues of concern to the teen with a disability, including dating, mobility, sexuality, and sports. Special sections on specific disabilities, with suggestions for school and other participation and a section on career planning.

10

Health Care

Most of us have had experience in obtaining medical care for ourselves or members of our family when we have had an illness or injury. Some of the same procedures will be used in obtaining care for your child with a chronic disability, but some additional and different steps are needed for ongoing care, and this chapter will focus on them.

In virtually any kind of chronic disability, a primary-care physician such as a pediatrician should be an important part of the process—someone who knows you and your family over time, who can evaluate and compile reports and information and can direct you to specialized help as you need it. In most instances, however, where chronic lifelong disability (such as cerebral palsy, spina bifida, Down's Syndrome, or maternal rubella syndrome) is involved, the primary physican can provide only a small amount of the service that is needed. Your child will need evaluation and treatment from a number of different professionals, and that service is usually best obtained when those professionals work in an interdisciplinary team setting, where they are accustomed to taking into account the findings of other specialists and tailoring their services so that they fit those provided by others.

*   *   *

The interdisciplinary team required by your child will be composed of specialists in those areas in which she requires help. It could include any or all of the following: occupational therapist, physical therapist, social worker, nurse, psychologist, special educator, speech and language pathologist, audiologist, nutritionist, geneticist, dentist. In addition to your pediatrician or other primary-care physician it may include medical specialists such as a neurologist, orthopedist, ophthalmologist, otologist, urologist, or cardiologist. At any given time, any one member of the team—the physical therapist, psychologist, speech pathologist, or neurologist, for example—may be giving the major amount of direct service, while other treatments are continued on a routine basis or even temporarily discontinued. Periodic evaluation (say yearly) should be done by all team members, however, and coordination of the various parts of your child's treatment program should be a continuing process.

Coordination is a necessary part of any treatment program that consists of different services provided by different specialists for different problems. It needs to be done by someone who has access to all of the information, can understand it well enough to see how the various parts relate to one another, and has the time to carry it out. If your primary-care physician can take the time to do the coordination, that is an excellent solution, although it may not be reasonable to expect the primary physician to have that amount of time available. Sometimes another member of the interdisciplinary team, such as a social worker or physical therapist, can do the major amount of coordination. There is one person who is ordinarily in a good position to be coordinator and who usually must play some part regardless of who is doing the job, and that is you, the parent.

Coordination may actually be thought of in several parts. Some of it is quite straightforward and practical: keeping track of all the appointments; straightening it out when, say, both OT and psychology appointments are scheduled for the same hour on the same days; planning for transportation to be available; caring for younger siblings while parents are consulting with professionals; and seeing that plans are not made for things like surgery and speech camp during the same week. Some parts of coordination are more subtle, such as noting that the nutritionist is suggesting a 1,000 calorie diet at the same time the physical therapist is instituting a very demanding exercise routine, or seeing that the ophthalmologist who wants to prescribe a drug is aware of the drugs already prescribed by the neurologist. Some coordination is a matter of arriving at priorities; for example, is the exercise of walking with braces more important than the efficiency and social acceptability of the wheelchair? Susan had been shy and friendless in high school. With some encouragement from the psychologist she joined a school club, began to help with its activities, and made a few friends. This coincided with a shift from half crutches and occasional use of an old wheelchair to regular use of a brand-new chair that she could propel rapidly. Soon Susan became a fixture in the halls, going back and forth and talking to people. The physical therapist became concerned about lack of exercise and suggested giving up the chair. Susan and the psychologist called for a conference that included Mom, the primary-care physician, and the physical therapist. The decision was that Susan's social gains and activities and good feeling about herself depended a great deal on getting around easily (and gracefully) in the chair and that she should go on using it. Her activities and growing sense of self continued to where she wanted to take care of herself physically. She asked for additional adaptive physical education and also looked out for opportunities to walk on her crutches. In the end, with her much larger schedule of activities, she was getting as much exercise as she had in the past, before she began to rely on the chair.

Certain aspects of coordination require the attention of the primary-care physician, who should be aware of the initiation of any major new treatment program and of the prescription of drugs or surgery. The primary-care physician should also be involved when there is a major difference of opinion about treatment among members of the treatment team, as was the case with Susan.

Much of the job of coordination can be done by you the parent, including calling needs to the attention of the physician and others. You should do as much of the coordinating job as you are capable of and available for. Eventually your child should begin to take over the coordination job for herself, beginning with remembering appointments, then calling to make appointments herself, and then on to more complicated matters. It is very important that you know that our health care system is not foolproof and that you cannot assume that somehow coordination will happen even if no one is paying attention to it.

Your child may require health care in four major categories: 1) acute medical care, 2) developmental remediation, 3) maintenance therapies, and 4) monitoring.

* * *

Acute medical care is typically needed at the onset of the disability. If the disability is present at birth the medical care might be surgery, such as the repair of the spinal cord in spina bifida or the heart in coronary disease. If the disability occurs later, as in spinal cord injury, acute care will be needed at the time of the injury. It may be required during episodes of disability such as occur in hemophilia or seizure disorder. Your child may also need acute medical care for problems that afflict many of us, such as chicken pox or a bad case of the flu.

Developmental remediation is treatment that is needed to help your child maintain progress in skills that may be affected by her disability. For example, if her muscles are weak or uncoordinated, she may need special exercises or even equipment from the physical therapist in order to learn to walk. If she has impaired hearing, poorly coordinated muscles in tongue and jaw, or delayed mental development, she may require help from the speech and language pathologist to learn how to speak. A child who because of disability has had limited contact with peers may need help from the psychologist or social worker to develop social skills.

Maintenance therapies are those routine treatments that are needed to keep your child healthy and functioning. Regular injection of insulin in diabetes is one of the best known, and regular use of anticonvulsants such as Dilantin for control of seizures is another. Boys with hemophilia need to infuse blood products at the earliest signs of bleeding into joints so as to prevent severe bleeds. Children with cystic fibrosis need regular percussing to remove congestive material from the lungs.

Children with cerebral palsy may need certain exercises in order to keep joints flexible and muscles strong.

Many of the maintenance therapies are done in the home, and many of them (even complicated ones such as infusing blood products into veins) can be carried out by the family. The ability to do this without specialized medical assistance usually means greater freedom for the family, who are not bound to remain within easy reach of medical services and are thus free to go on extended trips, camping, and so forth. This freedom to travel and sense of independence, not to mention reduction in medical costs, usually makes participation in home treatment a desirable goal. Such programs also usually provide an increased opportunity for the child to participate in her own treatment. This should be done starting as early as possible with simple parts of the treatment, such as being aware when treatment is needed. It should continue so that by the early teen years the patient may be responsible for the entire process.

Maintenance therapies are ones that frequently involve a certain amount of inconvenience or pain. The more the young patient knows about her disability and the effect of the treatment, the less likely she is to blame the parent for that inconvenience or pain. In any event, there is no justification for allowing the patient to skip treatment because she doesn't like it. Perhaps she may do that when she is a self-responsible adult who understands the consequences of skipping treatment and can decide for herself whether avoiding the pain or inconvenience is worth it. Young children, who are not old enough to understand what the decison means, should not be allowed to decide they will go without treatment because they don't like it. It is the responsibility of the parent to make that decision for them.

*   *   *

Monitoring is required to detect problems known to arise routinely, such as decubiti in persons who use a wheelchair regularly or bladder infections in those with devices for control of urinary functions. It may also be necessary to guard against treatment side effects, such as disruption of kidney function, that may occur from the use of powerful drugs. It is necessary to track possible changes in level of hearing or vision. Monitoring may be necessary to detect recurring episodes of disease, such as multiple sclerosis. Finally, as your child grows and develops it is necessary to see that equipment such as wheelchairs and braces continues to function and fit properly. Additional information about health care can be found in a number of the books listed at the end of this chapter.

It has been mentioned earlier in this chapter that you the parent may be in the best position to coordinate the health care of your child. Your logical successor is of course the child herself. As she grows up she should be as informed about her disability and its care as her level of understanding will permit. By her teen years she should begin to assume a major portion of the responsibility, provided that her disability does not interfere with her ability to understand and make judgments. Eventually she should keep medical and other appointments on her own, and she should be encouraged to persist in expressing her needs and in seeking understanding of the information and recommendations she receives. Many teens (and adults) need support in dealing with physicians and other professionals with sufficient assertiveness so that the consultation is effectively carried out.

*   *   *

In providing health care for your child, you will quickly become aware of the importance of health insurance. Without some system for financing it, access to health care in the U.S. is extremely limited. You will need to become acquainted with the requirements of whatever health coverage you may have and to weigh the consequences for continued care when considering actions such as a change in employment or residence that may result in a change of health coverage.

Pain is an unfortunate occurrence that cannot always be prevented, either because it is part of the disability or part of its treatment. Children with cerebral palsy or spina bifida may have repeated painful surgery and periods of recovery. Children with hemophilia may experience pain with internal bleeding. Pain may be constant, as in juvenile rheumatoid arthritis. Children with malignancies experience pain with progression of the disease. Treatments may include distasteful medicines or injections.

Rule number one is not to expect your child to act as if there were no pain at all. The approach is more one of "I know it hurts a lot," "Yes, it sure does taste yucky, but..," "I know you feel bad. So would I," "I don't blame you for crying if it hurts, but..." Allow the child time to express her hurt and resentment (at the pain, the disability, fate) and bad feeling. Empathize, and even sympathize somewhat. Then ask her to control it, put up with it, do what needs to be done.

Rule number two is not to allow the child to skip the treatment because she doesn't like it. Do not accept personal responsibility as the cause of pain, and above all, do not allow the pain to become a bargaining chip for getting a privilege or getting out of some other responsibility. It is quite appropriate, following a difficult treatment, to give the child a period of rest or pleasurable activity. It is not appropriate to bargain for this in advance or to allow acceptance of treatment to become a means of getting out of an expected responsibility. To do so is to teach the child that her illness or its treatment is a means for manipulating others, which can have disastrous consequences in many areas of her life.

This chapter on health services cannot be concluded without mention of the need for physical fitness. Disabled children, even more than the nondisabled, are in need of the highest level of physical fitness attainable for them. By this we mean regular physical activity, proper diet, and an adequate amount of sleep. Programs of physical exercise can be carried out by persons in wheelchairs, by persons on crutches, and by those who cannot use hands or arms, as well as those who may have limited vision or hearing. The physical therapist is an excellent source of suggestions for such a program, especially if you have concerns about your child's limitations. Diet is also a matter of special concern. Children whose enjoyable experiences are limited may turn to eating as a source of pleasure, resulting in obesity, which then acts to further increase the limitations on their other enjoyable social and recreational experiences. The conclusion that it really doesn't matter because they can't do anything anyhow is an unnecessary prescription for defeat. Your pediatrician or a nutritionist can help you with an appropriate diet. Seek help from others, such as the psychologist, social worker, occupational therapist, or recreational therapist in developing a program that will put interest and activity into the life of your child.

SOURCES OF ADDITIONAL INFORMATION

Jones, M.L. *Home Care for the Chronically Ill or Disabled Child*. New Yorker: Harper & Row, 1983.
A medically oriented book about the care of the chronically ill child in the home, which includes sections on medical treatment, dressing, feeding, and toileting, as well as other topics of psychological and social concern.

Lindemann, J.E., ed. *Psychological and Behavioral Aspects of Physical Disability: A Manual for Practitioners*. New York: Plenum, 1981.
Discusses the psychological problems associated with thirteen chronic disabling conditions, including cerebral palsy, spina bifida, progressive muscle disorders, sensory impairments, and others. Also contains brief descriptions of the etiology, diagnosis, and treatment of each disability. Addressed primarily to health care professionals.

Lindemann, J.E. and S.J. Lindemann. "A Typology of Childhood Disorders and Related Support Services," *Childhood Disability and Family Systems*, ed., M. Ferrari and M.B. Sussman. New York: The Haworth Press, 1987.
Contains a useful checklist and description of the support services that may be required by disabled

children in six categories: family, medical, financial, educational, psychosocial, and vocational.

Weiner, F. *Help for the Handicapped Child.* New York: McGraw Hill, 1973.

This reference book lists many common handicaps and discusses them with regard to description, treatment, prognosis, therapies, tests, and services. For each condition, it defines the vocabulary usually used. It also includes information on community, state, and government services and on health plans and insurance.

11

Socialization and Recreation

Every life needs its moments of pleasure, so that socialization for the joy of companionship and recreation simply for fun would be justification enough for this chapter. Yet there is much more: social skills are needed to function successfully in most important areas of our lives, such as going to school, holding a job, or being a parent; and recreation can be a means of socializing as well as a way to develop a sense of personal competence.

Socialization begins between child and parent, with the exchange of smiles and coos and squeals and touches. It gradually extends to others, who are recognized by the child and who acquire names. He learns to identify strangers, at first to avoid them and later to cope with them. The more people with whom the child becomes familiar and comfortable, the more socialized he will be, at whatever age. It is important to continue to expand those contacts, and this point is emphasized because there may be difficulty in doing so and it may seem easier in the short run to keep the child at home. He may look different or talk funny or have difficulty getting around or be slow to comprehend. Keeping him with people who "understand" will mean that he won't learn ways of coping, won't develop some tolerance for being seen as different, and will expect others to do the understanding and coping rather than assuming some of that responsibility himself. (Incidentally, you don't have to have a disability to develop this problem; it happens to nondisabled children as well.) One of the keys in avoiding this situation is that a significant amount of socialization should take place away from the family and with persons of the same age, not adults.

You expand the child's circle by having him play with siblings and cousins, visit relatives and neighbors, go to nursery school, preschool, and kindergarten. He should learn to play with kids in the neighborhood, then at the Y, church, or Scouts. He should go to a summer camp.

As your child develops, you may find yourself (and him) wondering if he should seek some of his social and recreational activity with other disabled children. You may answer that question in part by looking at how he has been doing up to that point in the mainstream. Are there areas of recreation in which he has a chance of occasionally being the winner, of being chosen for the team early (not last), of accounting for himself well? Does he have general acceptance from most of the children, the possibility of genuine friendship with at least a few, and occasional inclusion in evening or weekend activities? If the answers are mostly affirmative, then mainstream socializing may be the way to go. Further questions about the possible advantages of socializing with other handicapped persons: Can he learn some things from them about ways of dealing with his disability? Does the group have access to special equipment, or does it play games with special rules that will make participation more enjoyable? Are there matters of mutual interest, such as feelings about being different, that he would like to discuss with them? In general, our experience has been that those disabled persons do best who can (and do) participate in activities both in the mainstream and with other persons who have handicaps. If you or your child avoid socializing with handicapped people because of the stigma, this should give you pause for reflection. Does that mean that you (or your child) have placed that stigma on your child's disability, that you see it as embarrassing or unacceptable? Some open discussion, and perhaps some time with a counselor experienced with persons with handicaps, might help all of you arrive at a more comfortable position with regard to disability.

Recreation begins as the child learns to play. He should be provided with stimulating things that move, have color, and make noise. Learning to amuse oneself is important, as is learning to play with others. The child should have ample time for both. Later, play involves more complicated toys, then games that may be played alone and with others. Learning to play games by the rules is important for socialization and for fun. Passive play like watching TV or reading can be instructive, entertaining, and relaxing. Some play, however, should be neither passive nor directed by a set of rules. It is important that the child learn to play with things that require initiative and imagination, such as building blocks, drawing materials, dolls, trucks, houses, tools, and that require the player to create his own activity.

As your child grows older, his recreation is likely to become specialized according in his interests and abilities. It might involve individual physical activity such as swimming, tennis, skiing, hiking, Ping-Pong, or bowling; or it might involve team sports such as baseball, soccer, basketball, or football. It may involve sedentary games and activities such as checkers, chess, bridge, collecting, or being an avid attender of sports events. It may involve creative activities such as painting, acting, or playing an instrument. It may involve holding an office or participating in a civic or social club. No avenue of participation should be ruled out without at least a try. There are quadriplegic cartoonists, one-legged skiers, mentally retarded tennis players, blind cyclists, cerebral palsied wrestlers, and basketball players with spina bifida. There are adaptations, special groups, and forms of activity just waiting out there to be invented. Many can be discovered through organized groups such as the Special Olympics, National Wheelchair Athletic Association, Shared Outdoor Adventure Recreation (SOAR), U.S. Association for Blind Athletes, and public parks and recreation programs. Others can be found in the programs that are organized as part of disability groups such as United Cerebral Palsy, Association for Retarded Citizens, Spina Bifida Association of America, and the National Easter Seal Society. The names of other organizations, as well as further suggestions about recreation and leisure activities, can be found in a number of the books listed at the end of this chapter and at the end of Part I.

Recreation is important for fun. Recreation is important for socialization. Recreation can also play an extremely important role if it becomes the source of a person's feeling of special competence. Everyone likes and needs to have an area in which he has some special skill, knowledge, and achievement, whether it be a physical skill, an unusual collection, knowledge about rocks, perfect attendance at home games of the basketball team, ability to play cribbage, expertise at tying flies, or memorizing all the batting averages in the National League. Recreation is not the only area in which persons can develop a sense of competence. Many do it in their jobs or social activities. Recreation is an important area of accomplishment, and having a sense of competence in *some* area is vital to the development of self concept, the sense of *who I am*. One young woman has nicely combined many of her social, recreational, and vocational needs. Esther has moderate cerebral palsy and was only modestly successful as a high school student. She is energetic, personable, and outgoing, however, and has an abiding interest in outdoor recreation. Finding herself frustrated in attempts to prepare for a conventional career in sales or bookkeeping, she turned to her areas of strength and interest. She has forged a successful career as organizer and guide of outdoor expeditions for both disabled and nondisabled persons. She grins and says, "I get to have my cake and eat it, too."

Both recreational and social skills are important enough that steps should be considered for teaching them if necessary. Because persons with disabilities frequently start at a competitive disadvantage causing them to feel uncomfortable and embarrassed, it may be useful in some instances to carefully teach a skill. This could be in areas where training has traditionally been available, such as music, bridge, art, skiing, golf, or tennis. It can, however, also be in areas such as checkers, Ping-Pong, rummy, or even board games such as Monopoly or Parcheesi. Where the teen, whether because of shyness or ineptitude, has extra difficulty in learning such skills, the investment in special pretraining may be worthwhile. In some instances the activity may be, by choice or necessity, one that is primarily sedentary, such as collecting (stamps, rocks, coins, arrowheads), or it may even be a spectator activity, such as regular attendance at the games of a basketball, hockey, or baseball team. Any of these can become a valuable basis for the interactions that go on to become friendships, which generally need some activity, some grist for the mill, if they are to happen. In addition to recreational skills, social skills may be taught; frequently this is done in groups that are offered as part of a psychological or social service program. You can do some social-skill learning at home, by practicing what to say when you are introduced and how to make small talk, as well as the usual *please* and *thank you* amenities.

For a seriously disabled person to have something that approaches a normalized social and recreational life will frequently require a great deal in the way of support services. Transportation is the most common area of concern, and you should make every effort to make it available as readily as possible. This will involve the use of the family car or van, pooling with others, and use of public transportation. Your child will have a great advantage if he is eventually able to use the regular public transportation system or to drive a car. Communication is another necessary support system; learning to use the telephone at an early age, and having one available, can give a boost to socializing. Finally, children must have a place to get together at home, school, church youth center, Y, or commercial places such as movies, recreation centers, or restaurants.

When your child enters the teen years, he will need as much liberty as is appropriate to his maturity and judgment to come and go and be able to get together with his friends with some element of privacy. Disabled teens are not much different from others in their desire to get together, in having a great need for acceptance from peers and freedom from parents, and in their need to show individuality and independence by dress or actions that are, to some degree, outrageous. There is no real reason to expect disabled teens to be any more conforming or pious or placid than others, and always taking into account any special limitations in physical capacity or judgment, they should be treated no differently from their nondisabled siblings.

SOURCES OF ADDITIONAL INFORMATION

Hale, G., ed. *The Source Book for the Disabled: An Illustrated Guide to Easier, More Independent Living for Physically Disabled People, Their Families and Friends.* New York: Bantam, 1981.
A comprehensive how-to book with sections on daily living skills, leisure and recreation, sexuality, and other relevant topics. Includes an extended list of resource organizations and publications.

Levine, S.P., et al. *Recreation Experiences for the Severely Impaired or Non-Ambulatory Child.* Springfield, IL: Charles C. Thomas, 1983.
A how-to book that includes sections on movement activities, arts and crafts, music and listening activities, tactile and sensory activities. Sections on parent, family, and recreation with siblings. Appendix with sources of adapted equipment.

12

Sex and Marriage

It is a surprise to some parents to discover that their handicapped child is becoming a sexually interested young adult. Despite a body that is maturing in physical growth and function, it seems easy to expect a continued innocence and sometimes shocking to find it isn't there. This is part of the stereotyped way of looking at disability many of us share, and it can represent one more obstacle in the path of maturity and a normalized life. The truth is that virtually all disabled persons have sexual feelings, impulses, and desires. Most are capable of some manner of ordinary sexual activity, and for those few who are physically incapable of that, there are usually alternative approaches to sexual functioning that offer a high degree of stimulation and satisfaction as well as the opportunity to express love and affection. For persons who are very severely disabled, sexual stimulation may be one of a very limited number of available ways to feel good. Sexual activity for the person with disability, then, is not so much a matter of *if*, but rather *how, where, when,* or *with whom.*

Learning and practicing social skills is a necessary first step toward an eventual sexual relationship. One ordinarily begins with an acquaintanceship, which may become a friendship with mutual attraction and which may develop into a sexual relationship. In order to develop friendships, one learns skills such as what to say when you meet someone, how to make small talk, and what to do on casual contacts or dates. Some unfortunate incidents may occur when a person whose knowledge of socializing and sexuality comes from fantasy, locker room tales, or sex magazines decides it is time to have sex. Frequently the result is advances that are inappropriate and that lead to rejection, frustration, or more serious social consequences.

Parallel with the development of social skills should be sex education. This should begin early in your child's life, with information provided at home. The opportunity for this will usually occur with questions such as "Where did I come from?" or "Why is Mommy getting fat?" Such questions should be given answers that are simple, brief, and at a level appropriate to the age and understanding of the child. Most sex education at home should occur in small bits and pieces rather than in lengthy birds and bees lectures. Sex education should include precautions about advances and "bad touching" by strange or familiar persons. Children with disability are as likely to encounter sexual abuse as are others.

Some formal sex education given by an experienced person with the aid of books, pictures and other resources is highly desirable for most children, including those with a disability. This may be available in the school, through community service agencies, or through religious organizations. It should include information about the physiology of sexual functioning, how a child is conceived, and the possibility of family planning. Knowledge of safer-sex methods that control disease transmission has become a public health necessity for all of us in this time of the spreading AIDS (Acquired Immunodeficiency Syndrome) epidemic.

Sex education should always be presented in a context of interpersonal regard and responsibility. Children should learn, for example, that sex should not be used as a means of exploiting others or of allowing oneself to be exploited. They should also learn that it is a desirable and enjoyable part of a total relationship.

Your child, or you as parents, may have unanswered questions about sexuality that are related to disability and that might best be taken to professionals who are familiar with both disability and sexuality. Such questions might be: Is the person capable of ordinary sexual functioning (can the male have an erection, for example)? Is the person fertile? Does the disability have known genetic characteristics? Can it be inherited, and if so, what is the usual pattern of inheritance? Such information may be obtained from a number of professionals: physician, genetics counselor, nurse, social worker, or psychologist. It may be available through crippled children's services, disability-related associations, or private practitioners. It is usually helpful to set up separate appointments for discussing these matters so that both parents and the disabled person will have an opportunity to ask forthright questions and to discuss the matter frankly.

In discussing the interpersonal context of sexual relationships, many sex education programs use examples of appropriate and inappropriate behavior. This is particularly useful in working with persons of limited mental ability but also valuable in working with others, especially younger children. "It is appropriate to take off clothes in the bedroom but not in the kitchen." "Picking your nose in public is not appropriate." "You may rub yourself there in your bedroom, if you wish, but not in the living room." "A passionate embrace (if both parties agree) may be appropriate in private but not in the schoolyard." It may be necessary to point out some distinctions that seem very elementary, especially if the person has a limited ability to comprehend or has had limited social contacts.

The development of satisfactory sexual relationships may be more difficult for disabled persons for reasons that include the expectations set for them (to somehow be more innocent or virtuous than others); logistical difficulties (unavailability of transportation for getting to social events, lack of privacy); and the reality that some persons may find them less attractive than others. The remedies for these problems are numerous: developing the expectation that their needs and behaviors will be similar to others their age; assistance in the form of transportation; appropriate clothing and financial support to pay for attendance at functions; provision of privacy; and exposure to a wide variety of persons, disabled and nondisabled, with whom they might find mutual attraction.

Sexual intimacy is the logical extension of a loving and caring relationship, and the possibility of establishing a satisfying sexual relationship should not be dismissed casually. Given an available partner, persons with a wide variety of disabilities have been able to achieve such relationships. This may involve planning and willingness to experiment with different approaches. Problems such as incontinence can be managed with proper planning and arrangements. The possibility of pregnancy can be reduced with birth control methods. In some instances, aids may be useful in promoting sexual gratification. Even in cases where orgasm is physically impossible, disabled persons may experience an enjoyable "psychological orgasm" as the culmination of stimulating and gratifying their partner. The couple may need to work at combatting attitudes (held by themselves and others) that planning sex is unacceptable or that the use of aids or different approaches is kinky. Couples who have difficulty in developing a satisfying approach to sexuality may wish to consult a knowledgeable professional as well as some of the helpful books that are listed at the end of this chapter.

Being able to experience sexual gratification is one thing. Being able to conceive a child is another. Being married is something else. And being able to be successful at parenting is something else again. Most disabled persons can experience some level of sexual gratification. Many are also capable of sustaining a marriage relationship, and such a relationship can add a depth of meaning to a life that might otherwise be somewhat isolated. In addition to a caring relationship, a couple needs access to the physical capacity and skills to keep up a home, the judgment to make necessary decisions, and the ongoing financial support to pay the bills. Some or all of these factors may come from the couple themselves, and some (such as financial support or consultation about decisions) may come from elsewhere, providing it is reliably available over time.

Being married and being capable of sex does not necessarily mean that a couple is prepared to be parents. The matter of having children is an important question that should be substantially settled before marriage. It involves not only the stress of parenting on the individuals and the marriage but, most importantly, the ability to provide adequate parenting skills for the care of a child, including not only physical care but teaching and intellectual stimulation as well as the ability to cope with a variety of needs and emergencies as they arise. Some disabled persons are quite capable of highly successful parenting and should include children in their plans. Others who can adequately care for themselves and a marital partner may not have the skills that are necessary for successful child rearing, and in fairness to children, should not attempt to do so. That can be a difficult judgment to make, as the need to be parent and to "have something of my own to love and to love me" can be strong.

Jill and Kurt, who have been married for two years, complement each other in many ways. Jill is mildly retarded mentally and Kurt has moderate to severe cerebral palsy. He can get about without a wheelchair but is limited in physical strength, coordination, and dexterity. Jill is strong and clever with her hands but doesn't know enough arithmetic to follow recipes or keep a checkbook. Jill works in a hospital kitchen and Kurt in a sheltered workshop. Between them they manage a comfortable efficient household. They have a close relationship and an active sex life. They could have children but are still trying to decide if they can parent a child well enough to meet their own standards and if they want the stress that would be added to managing their lives. Jill's parents think they should not have children. Jill and Kurt are using birth control methods and have told themselves that they should decide within three years, since Jill is now twenty-seven.

In approaching marriage, couples that include a person with a disability may want to seek professional consultation together with regard to sexual functioning, the possibility of having children, and information about any known genetic characteristics of the disability.

SOURCES OF ADDITIONAL INFORMATION

Cornelius, D.A., et al. *Who Cares? A Handbook on Sex Education and Counseling Services for Disabled People*, 2nd ed. Baltimore: University Park Press, 1982.
This book has sections for professionals and for disabled persons. Several useful chapters dispel myths about sexuality and disability, answer basic questions about sex and marriage for the disabled person, and suggest sources of sex education and counseling.
Mooney, T.A., et al. *Sexual Options for Paraplegics and Quadriplegics*. Boston: Little, Brown, 1975.
Explores alternate and modified approaches to sexual interaction. Illustrated. For mature readers. (Contains graphic photographs.)

13

Vocation

Vocation plays a significant part in people's lives for a number of different reasons. Often it represents that area of special knowledge or competence around which they build their personal identity. It is what people frequently say when they finish the sentence "I am...," thinking of themselves as a bookkeeper, a repairman, a waitress, or a teacher. It may be a total or partial means of financial support. It frequently provides an important framework about which people organize their lives: a reason for getting up, for getting dressed, and for going out into the world. It can play these roles whether it is full-time or part-time, in the competitive world of work or in a sheltered setting.

Preparation for vocation has been going on throughout the life of your child as she has learned adaptive behavior and social skills. In order to function in the vocational world, one must be able to get to work, to care for her own needs during the day, and to get along with her supervisors and fellow workers. More jobs have been lost through lack of social skills (inability to get along with others) than through lack of work skills. Saying hello and good-bye, giving eye contact when addressed, and acknowledging that you have heard an instruction are things that may not be written in job descriptions and in fact may not be mentioned as reasons for terminating a person's employment. They are, however, frequent underlying reasons for an employer's conclusion that a person is unsuitable. Learning these social skills is ordinarily not directly impeded by disability. It is not realistic to expect a person to manage herself independently in a work setting if she has not been able to do so at home, in school, or elsewhere. So the first thing that needs to be done when the person begins to think seriously about job preparation is to survey those everyday skills she will need to get there and to maintain the job. Sometimes some additional homework is needed.

Among the important growing-up experiences are some that have a direct relationship to work. These include chores at home, which should be simple in the beginning, become more complex, and eventually involve a sustained period of effort as well as the requirement that the one who does the chores be personally responsible for knowing when they need to be done and for initiating them. Part-time or summer work such as lawn mowing, babysitting, store clerking, or fast food service also can represent very useful preparation for a later career, if such jobs are available and do not interfere with school. Many high schools have work experience programs that are part of the curriculum, and a number of federally funded community programs may offer summer work experience. In the absence of paid employment, work as a volunteer can also be very useful in developing vocational skills.

Work experience in various settings can help a person arrive at a realistic knowledge of what employment is about and of their capacity to do it. Achieving this

represented a problem for Mary Lou. She was nineteen, a
high school graduate in a wheelchair because of spina
bifida. She came for vocational assistance, saying that all
she needed was to get a job, as she had clerical skills
and in fact was working at a regular job in her father's
print shop. Detailed discussion revealed that she worked
at her father's business about three hours per day,
answering the telephone, typing the messages, and occasionally addressing envelopes. She was typing fifteen
words per minute. Mary Lou got very upset at the
suggestion that this was not the equivalent of full-time
clerical employment. She persevered, however, and over
several months she was seen twice monthly for counseling sessions and her working hours were extended. She
then went into six months of business school training,
which was arranged by the Vocational Rehabilitation
Division (see pages 141–142). Her feelings of competency
increased as did her knowledge of the world of work.
Today she is happily employed in a full-time job in a down-
town business office. The self-confidence she developed
in the vocational world has also helped her in the decision
to move from the family home to a shared apartment.

Vocational preparation may also involve some school
choices. Plans for four-year college should include the
scheduling of college preparatory courses during the
high school years. A person whose career will be built
on nonacademic skills may need greater emphasis on
practical or vocational experiences during high school.

Toward the end of the school years your child should
begin to narrow her career goals, basing her choices on
those activities she likes to do (interests) and those
things she is able to do (abilities). Sometimes this
narrowing or focusing occurs naturally, as a result of
experiences in everyday life: chores, hobbies, social ex-

periences, and school studies, as well as knowledge of vocations gained from reading or the media. The person may have done her own job of learning about herself and about the world of work. Many people, with or without disability, need some help in the form of vocational evaluation and career counseling in order to sort out those possibilities that fit with their interests and abilities. They may not know the work components or the skills required for a job in which they are interested. They might not know if their abilities are sufficient to cope with a certain course of training or to do a certain kind of work. They may have difficulty in translating their hobbies, recreational pursuits, academic preferences, and social activities into job interests. They may not know if there is a market for a certain kind of skill or if training programs are available for them. For them, vocational evaluation and career counseling can be invaluable.

Some evaluation and counseling is available through many public school programs. School counselors are usually good sources of information about colleges, college entrance, scholarships, requirements, and procedures. The evaluation methods used in the schools may be of limited usefulness in making decisions among technical, blue-collar, or entry-level jobs. In many schools the student is given group instruction about the meaning of tests taken, with limited individual assistance in interpreting results. Most schools do not provide the individualized evaluation of abilities that is needed when the person has a serious impairment of hearing, vision, or physical dexterity. They may or may not have available a career counselor who is experienced in working with people with disabilities.

In some states, vocational evaluation and career counseling are offered through the crippled children's service, and such services can also be useful sources of referral if they do not offer the counseling themselves. Vocational evaluation and career counseling are also offered as a service by some commmunity colleges and universities. In addition, they may be obtained through private psychologists or counselors. The person you see should have appropriate professional credentials plus experience in working with persons who have disabilities. An experienced evaluator is especially important if your teen's handicap is such that it will influence her ability to take tests or carry out certain functions in future employment. The Vocational Rehabilitation Division in your state will offer vocational evaluation and counseling when you are accepted by them for active services. This may be your primary source of evaluation and counseling unless these services are required for decisions early in the person's high school career. In that case, it may be necessary to obtain them from the sources mentioned above.

The Vocational Rehabilitation Division (VRD) is an agency supported by federal and state funds that may be found in every state. Its mission is to prepare persons with disabilities to become employable and employed. Most states have a separate agency, commonly called the Commission for the Blind, to serve persons who are legally blind. These agencies are available to all; there are no residence or financial requirements for eligibility, although some services, such as payment for training programs, treatment, or vocational tools, may be based on financial need. VRD offers services to evaluate abilities as well as physical or mental disabilities. In some instances it will provide treatment services to help a person become employable. It offers counseling to choose an appropriate vocational goal. It will provide training as needed, in settings ranging from the sheltered workshop to vocational schools or universities. In some instances it will provide the person with the tools of the trade, such as mechanic's equipment. It will offer assistance in job finding. If you have a significant disability you should investigate the services of VRD, regardless of your financial circumstances and regardless of whether you need help in choosing a goal. The agency can frequently add helpful support services and advice. VRD is an especially good source of knowledge about the training opportunities in your locality, particularly regarding community colleges, trade schools, business schools, allied health, on-the-job, and other specialty training.

Vocational evaluation should help a person to decide the *direction* of her career based on her interests as measured on tests and also as seen in her choice of hobbies, sports, school functions, and social activities. Are her interests mechanical, scientific, artistic, in business, sales, or other services to people? Evaluation should also help the person to decide the *level* at which she will aim, based on measures of abilities as well as on past successes (or failures) in activities and in school courses. In most areas of interest a person can work at an entry level with little training, at a technical level, or at the level of a professional or manager. In science one can be a physicist, an electronics technician, or an electronics assembly worker. In business one can be a CPA, a sales representative, a retail clerk, or a shelf stocker. Most vocational goals will require training beyond that available in the public school (usually a good investment for the disabled person, anyhow). Training may be obtained in a four-year college, in community college, in vocational or business school, on the job, or in a sheltered setting. The vocational goal should be in an area that interests the person and at a level at which she is capable of functioning. It should use skills that she has or that she will be able to learn.

If there is a serious question of the person's long-range ability to do college-level work, then evaluation is appropriate early in the high school years so that college preparatory courses can be scheduled if that does become her goal. In any event, a prospective four-year-college student should have formed at least tentative career plans one year before finishing high school so as to allow for the timely completion of college applications. In other instances, the question may be whether it will be of benefit for a person to continue to work primarily on academic subjects during high school or whether attention might better be given to practical or vocational skills. Again, this would suggest the value of early evaluation and counseling. In many other instances, however, evaluation during the last year of high school will suffice, as is also true in most cases where the intention is to pursue training in a community college, a business or vocational school, entry-level employment, or a sheltered setting.

For persons of limited ability or severe disability, or those who have very limited social skills or work experience, a sheltered setting may be the place to begin. Sheltered workshops allow the person to try different jobs, to learn specific job skills (sometimes very technical ones), and to develop sound work habits. Persons even more severely disabled may get similar experience in a work activity center. Other sheltered opportunities may also be available, such as in enclaves (where groups of handicapped persons work with the help of a trainer), subsidized work positions, or supported employment.

Some persons have unnecessarily negative stereotypes about sheltered workshops. If such a setting is suggested for your young adult, you are strongly urged to become directly acquainted with the sheltered setting before forming an opinion or making a judgment. A visit or, better yet, a trial experience in a sheltered setting will frequently reveal that it is more supportive, pleasant, and productive than had been imagined. We have had a number of positive experiences in which disabled persons were able to get a four-to-six-week evaluation in a sheltered workshop during the summer before their senior year of high school. The result has usually been a much more favorable attitude toward sheltered workshops, as well as increased self-knowledge. Be sure to ask about the workshop's record of training and employment. Sheltered settings are especially good for helping the person to develop positive work habits and to eliminate negatives ones. Positive habits include getting there on time, ability to persist at a task, and pride in a job well done. Some common negative problems are talking and socializing that interferes with others and behaviors that are grossly inappropriate and disruptive.

The final vocational step is obtaining the job. The Vocational Rehabilitation Division and some other community programs can offer valuable *assistance* with this, helping the person to organize a job hunt and helping to plan and rehearse how to present herself to an employer on paper (through the résumé) or in person. In a few instances it may be appropriate for a placement specialist to intervene where it is important to inform the employer about the nature of the disability or to suggest ways of modifying the job so a person with a disability can do it. When it is a job in the competitive labor market, however, nothing can replace the presence and commitment of the potential employee herself. The reality of competitive employment is that it cannot be achieved without the involvement of the individual, who must want it and seek it. No agency can do the entire placement for you. In fact, the realistic prescription for becoming employed is to work at it full-time and to present yourself to a number of possible employers every day. This, rather than through agencies, is the way most persons become employed.

In some instances, because of the severity of disability or other circumstances, the prospect is for a person to be engaged in long-term employment in a sheltered workshop or activity center. In most cases this is far superior to staying at home. It provides a focus for daily activity, opportunity for socializing, a change of scene for the employee, relief for those at home, and usually some, albeit limited, financial return. It usually means that the person will continue to improve in potential rather than regress because of idleness. In some instances people make the transition to regular employment after many years in a sheltered setting. Such a sheltered setting can be a significant part of a life, along with the other social and recreational activities that round it out.

SOURCES OF ADDITIONAL INFORMATION

Lobodinski, J., et al. *Marketing Your Abilities: A Guide for the Disabled Job-Seeker.* Washington, D.C: Mainstream, Inc., 1984.

A brief pamplet that describes the job search, including self-assessment, preparation of a résumé, the interview, and coping with rejection.

Mitchell, J.S. *See Me More Clearly: Career and Life Planning for Teens with Physical Disabilities.* New York: Harcourt, Brace, Jovanovich, 1980.

Discusses issues of concern to the teen with a disability, including dating, mobility, sexuality, and sports. Special sections on specific disabilities, with suggestions for school and other participation, and a section on career planning.

14

Where to Live

Where your child with a disability will live during his childhood is not generally a matter of unusual concern or discussion. In most instances he will live in the parental home. Living at home may not be uncomplicated, of course, as it may involve installing ramps or other adaptive equipment. Where disability is especially severe, where it requires specialized services, or where there are other demands on the family, it may mean that outside help will be needed at times. In a few instances the child will be in an institutional setting.

It is when your child approaches young adulthood, the time for moving out into the world, that the issue of where he should live may become a matter of concern. There are many reasons moving out is the usual pattern for young adults. It is a time when they are trying to become a person in their own right, to have an identity that is not a carbon copy or an extension of their parents'. It is a time when parents may want the time and freedom from responsibility that will allow them to pursue their own interests. Patterns of control and dependence do not change easily for parents or for children, and a bit of distance helps.

The options open to your child will depend a great

deal on the extent to which he can care for himself.
Disability may play a major role: Can he get about home
and community on his own? Does he have the manual
dexterity for self-care, including cooking, doing household
repairs, and so forth? Does he have the reasoning ability
and judgment to manage himself in a household? How well
he has incorporated the attitudes of independence and the
skills of daily living at home will also play a major role.

Residence in a *group home* is a frequent first step for
the disabled young adult who has been living with
parents. It can be a valuable transition experience, giving the young person the opportunity to learn to care for his
own room and belongings, to share household duties
such as cooking and cleaning, and to handle a large
degree of responsibility for his own hours and activities.
It provides the opportunity to work and to socialize with
peers, which is especially useful if that has been limited
in the past. It may provide some specialized services,
such as assistance from a nurse, social worker, or therapist. Group homes differ in the support services and
degree of supervision they provide and should be investigated individually with regard to their suitability for
your young adult. Some are set up for long-term residence and some for transition periods. Visits for a day or
a weekend are useful ways to become acquainted with
the group home, its services, and its rules.

Another step in the direction of independent living
for the young adult who has had group home experience,
or who does not need that transition, is living in a
satellite apartment. Where these are available, they are
often run by service organizations such as associations
for people with cerebral palsy or mental retardation.
They are sometimes run in conjunction with group
homes. They are apartments for two to four persons,

usually all of whom have some degree of disability, who share the rent as well as the responsibility for cooking, cleaning, and their own self-care. Remote supervision may be provided by a staff person who lives nearby and is available for emergencies, assistance with major purchases, consultation on routine problems such as menus or simple repairs, and occasional on-site visits. While there may be some difference in contribution of skills, with one more experienced in shopping, another in cleaning, and yet another in cooking, each person is basically responsible for meeting his own needs or for working out arrangements with others to do so.

Many persons with disability are quite capable of *totally independent living.* They may live by themselves, with roommates or spouse, in an apartment or house, with full responsibility for its operation. Sometimes this is done with a circumscribed amount of support, such as the service of an attendant who may appear once or twice a day to assist with particular functions such as bathing, toileting, or dressing. Some persons can function independently with only the occasional availability of others to help in matters such as finding housing, making a major purchase, or signing a contract.

The timing of the move from the parents' home is an important matter. Certainly it is appropriate for a young person to stay at home while completing education, commuting to school, or returning home during holidays and vacation periods. It may be appropriate for the young adult to live at home briefly while beginning a job, affording the opportunity to make one adjustment at a time as well as to save a nest egg for the independent start. In general, however, it is best to plan for the young adult to move out soon after the completion of his schooling. For many, the experience of dealing with peers and being self-responsible is necessary if they are to become truly independent. For some it may be a difficult experience, but it will ordinarily best be done while they are relatively young and have some degree of flexibility. The parents as well as the young person will generally suffer if the parent-child dependency relationship is maintained until circumstances force its end. If the reasons for postponing a move are along the lines of "No one else understands him," "He won't eat anyone else's cooking," or "He raises a ruckus with anyone else," it is time to be concerned and to make a plan for transition while you as parents are young enough to be helpful in carrying it out and the disabled person is young enough to adapt to it. It may be necessary to get professional help from a psychologist or social worker in setting up such a plan.

The transition to another place of residence is usually not without some discomfort during the adjustment period. Old habits and old relationships are broken, and new ones formed. It takes time, and it is ordinarily best to allow plenty of time for the transition to take place. First attempts may fail or may work for a while and then require change. The person should know that he is loved and is not being rejected, but should also not be encouraged to run home when frustrations occur. That being said, however, it should also be pointed out that moving out does not mean the end of old relationships. Visits can and should occur—on holidays and during vacation periods. The young adult can come home for Sunday dinner or birthdays. Some social and recreational activities (a show, ball game, dinner out) may also be shared with family if this is done after the individual has established an independent pattern of social and recreational activities and if this is not allowed to supplant those activities. In some instances these activities with the family may include the person's new friends. The final relationship with your young disabled adult should resemble that with any other member of the family who has gone out on his own.

In addition to group home, satellite apartment, or independent living, there are a number of other arrangements that may be considered under some circumstances. The *adult foster home* is an arrangement in which one or more persons live in a family setting. This is usually more supportive and more restrictive than group home living, with concomitant advantages and disadvantages. It will usually not provide as much peer contact as is found in the group home. Some persons, especially those in need of an extensive amount of assistance with self-care, may reside in *nursing homes*. These frequently allow for only a restricted amount of personal activity and may not, for example, allow a schedule that permits the resident to hold employment. Some nursing homes are set up primarily for young adults, but most cover a wide age range, with emphasis on older persons, and thus do not provide peer experiences for the young adult. In some instances, *residence in a hospital or other large institution* is required. Reasons for this are usually very severe physical disability or the presence of severe behavioral, social, or emotional disturbances that cannot be managed in other than a controlled environment. While conditions in such institutions have vastly improved in recent years and they generally provide a variety of social, recreational, and vocational experiences, they continue to represent a solution that is costly for society and restrictive of life satisfaction for their residents. For further discussion of institutional placement, see Chapter Seventeen.

Many of the residential programs discussed here have requirements for eligibility, procedures for application, and sometimes, very long waiting lists for entrance. You would be well advised to begin your planning early and to find assistance in doing so. Assistance is available from a variety of social service agencies, including your crippled children's service, developmental disabilities agencies, or the private agencies that provide support for many types of disabilities.

SOURCES OF ADDITIONAL INFORMATION

"Alternatives for Community Living." News Digest. Washington, D.C: National Information Center for Handicapped Children and Youth (April 1986).

Article describes various community-based living arrangements, including information on funding and respite care.

Roberts, S., and N. Sydow. *Consumer's Guide to Attendant Care.* Access to Independence, Inc.: Madison, Wisconsin, 1984.

A step-by-step guide for assessing the need for an attendant, advertising for, interviewing and hiring an attendant, training and utilizing the services of an attendant.

15

Advocacy

Advocacy means effective representation for a person or cause. Persons with disability may be in need of advocacy for a number of reasons: sometimes their needs, though real, are not obvious, and others may have to be persuaded that they should be met; sometimes they need services or facilities that do not presently exist, so that the resources must be mobilized, as well as others persuaded; and, finally, in these days of restricted budgets, agencies such as school districts and health care providers may need to be prodded to provide services that are already mandated. Some disabled persons can be their own advocates; some need assistance.

You should not be reluctant to speak up in seeking the proper services for your disabled child in your dealings with health care providers, schools, rehabilitation or other agencies. You should be sure that you carry out your advocacy with constructive assertiveness. A helpful way of promoting access to and experience with advocacy was devised in one school district by interested parents working with special education support personnel. A Parent-to-Parent group was formed by parents of children with disabilities (of all kinds). The group assembled information regarding numerous local and national organizations, including those that serve specif-

ic disability groups as well as those that provide
services such as transportation and recreation to a broad
range of persons with disability. The group contacts
parents of disabled children to inform them of the presence of the service and offers the option of as little or as
much participation as they wish. Parents can be put in
touch with a parent of a child with similar disability.
Parents can ask for an advocate to assist them in participation at IEP meetings (meetings to formulate and discuss Individual Education Programs). Or they may avail
themselves of source material to assist them in their
own learning and advocacy.

There are some guidelines for being constructive in
your advocacy. To begin with, you should take the initiative to communicate with the important people or groups
that serve your child and continue the communication
on a routine basis. In school, go to the classroom and
make a point of meeting the teacher. Be sure the school
is able to reach you in case of emergency, by providing
home and work phone numbers and notifying them if
they change. Go to school conferences. With your health
care personnel, keep appointments, ask questions, and
make sure both parents keep informed, preferably by
making appointments together or alternating the responsibility.

In some instances you will be dealing with large
agencies or with professionals who are part of a group.
They will have many patients, students, or clients. You
cannot wait for them to come to you. If you see a
problem or something you *think* is a problem, do something about it by pointing it out, asking for an appointment, asking for help. Do not be so polite or so hurt by
feeling rejected that you let the matter slide because

you don't want to make the next move. In some cases the agency or group has made a mistake and really should be dealing with the problem. Usually they will be happy that you brought it up, whether it turns out to be a major problem or not.

A theme that runs through all of this is that you need to be informed. Nothing can be a substitute for having an understanding of your child's condition and the treatment she is receiving. If you don't understand, ask questions. If you feel your ability to understand is limited, try to get help from someone you trust—a relative, a friend, or a professional with whom you feel you can communicate. Your ability to be an advocate will depend on your ability to understand. In most states, the designated advocacy agency can provide you with informational materials regarding your child's right to educational or health care services.

Some of your understanding may be attained through acting as coordinator for your child. Coordinating is itself a kind of advocacy and has been discussed elsewhere in this book (see Chapter Ten). Someone needs to keep track of appointments, see that they do not conflict, and make sure the child gets there. Someone needs to understand the recommendations so that they do not conflict—for example, that a new medication that may cause drowsiness is not started during exam week. Some of the coordination may be carried out by a professional such as a pediatrician or social worker. Some agencies, such as those for Mental Retardation/Developmental Disability (MR/DD), will provide some coordinating service. No one is likely to be able to coordinate with as personal a touch and as unique a knowledge of the child as you the parent. You should do as much of it as you are able. You will then be in an excellent position to be an advocate for your child.

In working with large agencies, it is helpful to learn enough about their organization so that you can contact the person in the decision-making position. This can be particularly important in the schools. For example, if your child is in a special program, then contact with the supervisor of that program, in addition to the child's teacher, will usually be necessary if important changes or additions are to be made. There may be similar relationships in health care programs when one person carries out services on the recommendation of another.

Finally, if you are to have a solid basis for your advocacy, you should be sure that what you expect for your child is realistic. If you see something as possible for your child, can you describe to others what it is that you see? If there is a difference of opinion, what do disinterested third parties think? Obtain opinions from others. Is the service you request available anywhere? And at what price? Are your hopes and desires for your child causing your expectations to be unrealistic? You can expect your child to have a medical, educational, or other program tailored to her unique needs. You cannot expect it to be set up as if she is the only child in the system, even if she is your only child.

So, you have set the stage to be a good advocate. You have been in communication with the appropriate parties, and you understand what is going on. You know to whom to direct questions and have done so. You believe that your expectations are realistic. The day may come when there is an honest difference of opinion about what your child needs, and that is the time for constructive assertiveness. You must state your opinion to the persons serving your child and to the supervisor of that program. You have your information at hand, know what you are requesting, and you express it forcefully, without too much emotion. You may need to appeal to the director of a service or organization, to its governing board, or even to elected officials. You may have to marshal professional opinions from third parties. You may wish to seek help from a support group that is related to your child's disability or from an advocacy agency. Part of P.L. 98–527 mandates that there shall be a protection and advocacy system in each state. If you have been in touch, understand the problem, and are asking for something realistic, the chances of success are excellent. Do it—and good luck.

One further word should be said about a kind of activity that goes beyond *personal* advocacy for your child. You should strongly consider joining an advocacy group that is related to your child's area of disability. In that way you can lend your weight to the effort to raise money, develop programs, and lobby for legislation that will be to the benefit of all members of that group, including your child. That participation should also make you a better personal advocate, one who is informed and who knows how to bring about change.

SOURCES OF ADDITIONAL INFORMATION

Haskins, J. and J.M. Stifle. *The Quiet Revolution: The Struggle for the Rights of Disabled Americans.* New York: Crowell, 1979.
Describes the birth of the disabled rights movement. Contains sections on the right to prevention of disability, treatment, education, employment and compensation, and a barrier-free environment.
Williams, P. and B. Shoultz. *We Can Speak for Ourselves: Self Advocacy by Mentally Handicapped People.* Bloomington: Indiana University Press, 1982.
Contains chapters on learning self-advocacy, developing a self-advocacy group, and a manual for self-advocacy. Has broad usefulness for people with many kinds of disabilities.

16

Children with Sensory Impairments

If you suspect that your child has a problem with seeing or hearing, the first thing you should do is seek competent evaluation. Assessing infants or very young children with sensory impairments is difficult, and you should seek the services of persons who are trained and experienced in dealing with problems of hearing or vision in this age group. You don't have to (and shouldn't) "wait and see" if you sense that your child has decreased vision or hearing. Specialized techniques have been developed to measure the levels of adequacy of these senses in very small children. In addition to these measures, your reporting about how your child reacts in situations in the home will be an important part of the assessment.

As in most problems, there is a range of severity to be found in sensory deficits. Your child may have a mild visual loss, or she may be blind. She may have a mild hearing loss, or she may be deaf. Some losses affecting our senses can be static (remain at the same level all our lives), and some can be progressive (get worse with age). Some can be treated medically or surgically. Some visual problems may be partially or totally corrected with glasses, and hearing may be improved with amplification (hearing aids). Early diagnosis is important so that a treatment plan or intervention plan can be started.

The need for early intervention in sensory deficits has to do with the importance of the senses in developing language and in communication. If your child sees or hears poorly, it decreases the amount of information she can take in and use in the process of learning. The child who is very nearsighted may be unable to get an idea of distance or the full size and detail of larger objects. The child who is blind is delayed in naming objects because she does not see them. She also cannot make use of common concepts, such as color, in description. The child who is hearing impaired may get only bits of the conversation going on around her and may not easily grasp the whole of what is being said. The child who is deaf must rely entirely on visual cues to interpret what is going on about her. So it is important to help your child early in her life to adopt alternative ways to taking in information. Unless this occurs early, your child may be seriously impaired in her ability to understand and develop language concepts.

Sometimes as a result of accident or illness, older children may be left with vision or hearing loss. This is particularly traumatic because these children are suddenly unable to communicate in a manner familiar to them and will experience the frustration of having to struggle to do things that came easily before and of being unable to do things for themselves that before they could. The newly blind child will have had some awareness of the form of the world about her. If your child should lose her hearing at an age after speech and language have been acquired, she will have the advantage of the basics, even though she may need to adopt alternative methods of receiving information. However, the effective loss of these senses will often have a powerful emotional impact on children (and families) and it may be necessary to devote even more attention to handling fears, frustrations, depression, and anxiety than is the case when disability is present from birth.

If your child has limited distance vision, you will want to make sure that you present things close enough for her to see before you expect her to react to them. If she can see in only a narrow range (in the middle or near the edges of her vision), you must then allow more time for her to scan the material. If she is blind, you will want to make early use of sounds for stimulation. Children who are blind tend to be somewhat delayed in motor development; this is probably because they are not motivated to move about toward things when they cannot see them. So a child who is blind may not crawl or respond to other people as soon as a child who has sight. It is *very* important to talk a great deal to children who are severely visually impaired or blind, describing what is around them and what is happening. Teach them to explore with their hands and to become familiar with shapes and textures. Teach them that cotton balls are soft and fluffy, that sandpaper is rough, and that boxes have corners and can be large. Later, when you describe clouds as being soft and fluffy, the sidewalk as being rough, and tall buildings as being like big boxes, your child will be able to understand the language concepts and use them to comprehend what she cannot see.

If your infant is severely visually impaired or blind, you should seek early intervention programs that are specialized in teaching such children. Teachers can give you ideas about how and what to teach your child in the home. In school, special devices and training may be made available, depending on need. Large print material may be employed as children go past the primary print used in the first few years of school. Magnification by various means may be appropriate and necessary. If your child will not be a print reader, the pre-Braille and Braille skills will need to be started. Touch typing, orientation and mobility training, and the use of taped materials are processes that can be introduced at appropriate times.

For the child who is blind, going about the community independently can be as anxiety-provoking (for parents and child) as it is desirable. Needless to say, it requires that the child have careful mobility training and an appropriate level of judgment. When these have been achieved, it is part of your responsibility to allow the child to go, and to be supportive as she goes through the early stages of this activity, which you will eventually value as important and rewarding for everyone involved.

An accommodation will need to be found between the child's individual needs and the minimum amount of equipment required. If she can get along with regular size print plus some magnification, this will greatly increase the amount of reading material readily available. Large print books are bulky, and the variety of material is more limited. In the long run, however, it is most important that materials that are appropriate are available and that your child (and you) learn how to use them. Your vision specialist teacher will have much helpful information about methods and materials, as well as information about such things as lighting and comfortable reading distance. Many children who are visually impaired, even when their vision is corrected as fully as possible, may need to hold reading materials close to their eyes and should be allowed to do so. There are many simple as well as very sophisticated pieces of equipment now on the market that can assist people who are visually handicapped. You should assure yourself that your child can make effective use of these devices before you invest in them. One way to do this is by asking a specialist in the field who is not engaged in selling such devices.

Hearing impairment in a child is not always recognized as early as visual impairment. If your child is hearing impaired she may be delayed in speech development, and when speech comes, it may be hard for you to understand. This is because she is not hearing all of the speech sounds well enough to learn how to imitate them and because she cannot hear herself well enough to hear how she sounds so that she can self-correct. This is why early intervention is so important for the development of both language (learning what words mean) and speech (how to say them). If hearing aids are recommended for your child, you should see that they are obtained, fitted, and monitored by an appropriate agency after she has had a medical evaluation. A qualified audiologist is needed to determine which amplification system best fits your child's needs. The audiologist can also advise you about methods for training the tiny child to accept and tolerate the aid. You will need to learn about maintenance of the aids and the molds (individualized plastic inserts fitted to the ear) and when and how to change batteries until your child is old enough to assume this responsibility herself.

Some kinds of hearing loss can be of short duration because they are caused by factors that can be corrected by medical treatment or surgery. Ear infections can cause hearing to be impaired on a short-term basis. These are usually relieved by medication or by surgically inserting tubes to drain the ears. Repeated ear infections can lead to some permanent hearing loss. For this reason it is important to treat ear infections whenever they occur. These temporary or conductive losses are usually not ones in which the use of hearing aids is recommended.

Other hearing losses may be due to illness or hereditary factors or to structural abnormalities present at birth. These are known as sensorineural losses, which include permanent damage to the inner ear or auditory nerve. Hearing aids are often recommended to improve the hearing of individuals with sensorineural loss.

After you have followed through with an appropriate amplification system for the child with a hearing loss, you should think about her communication and how it is limited—both receiving and sending. If she is deaf or severely impaired, the avenue of receiving through the ears is limited, and early training should emphasize visual methods of introducing material. When you talk to her, make sure she can see your face for speech reading (lip reading) and facial expression. The use of gestures with speech is a natural and appropriate way to give more bits of information to be received. Early intervention programs for the hearing impaired also provide techniques to assist your child in speaking as clearly as possible. Communication should be developed to its fullest to give the most opportunities for mainstream participation. The use of manual signing should be seen as a supplement to speech as well as a means for increasing language acquisition.

The question of the most effective method of communication for the deaf is a subject of continuing debate among those who believe that the Oral Method is best and those who believe the Total Communication Method is most appropriate. The Oral Method stresses development and use of residual hearing, speech reading, and speaking, while Total Communication includes elements of the Oral Method plus the use of gestures and manual signs. In considering the options for your child, you should seek information from all sources and be aware of the controversial nature of the issue. Seek advice from professionals, visit different kinds of classrooms, and talk with teenagers or adults who are deaf. Our feeling is that the best method is one that 1) provides a means for full and early language development both for receiving (receptive language) and sending (expressive language); 2) promotes speech development to its highest possible level; and 3) provides a *workable* method of communication between you and your child. If speech development and residual hearing are clear enough, the Oral approach may be appropriate. However, if your child cannot hear adequately to understand speech and if you cannot understand what she says, then manual signs should supplement the speech training. It is very important that language concepts and vocabulary building start early and a method by which you and she can *do* this should be started early. As with any disability, do only what is necessary to promote an ordinary or mainstream method, but don't deny your child a means of communication.

With either type of sensory impairment, the same general approaches to behavior and independent functioning apply. There should be the same expectations for self-care and behavior as for nondisabled children, making allowance only for the things they obviously cannot do. Barry is a child whose condition of blindness from birth caused much disruption in the family. From infancy, things were done for him and he was allowed to have his way, with few or no limits on his conduct. At age ten he controls the family with tantrums and destructive behavior. In contrast, Lila's blindness from birth was met in such a way that expectations for her behavior and learning were no different from those of her siblings. She was given much verbal stimulation, and she was expected to dress and feed herself as soon as was physically possible. She was disciplined when she misbehaved and praised for her accomplishments. At age seven she is an inquisitive and self-assured child. The way Avis was reared by her family demonstrates this even further. For example, as a totally blind (from birth) twelve-year-old she rode her bicycle all over their quiet suburban neighborhood. She did this with the aid of her younger sister, who rode her bicycle one length in front of Avis's, with a noisemaker inserted in the spokes. (The noisemaker provided indication of increase or decrease in speed, as well as a signal to follow.) As an adult, Avis looks back and laughs, "People used to think the things my parents did to me were outrageous. Sometimes I did. They couldn't have done it better. I guess I learned to try harder."

Your child who is vision impaired or hearing impaired should have responsibility for self-care and other chores. If equipment such as glasses or hearing aids is to be worn, its use should be consistent and responsibility for this should be taken over by the child when age-appropriate. A word about glasses and hearing aids: they do a child little good if their use is limited to clinic visits or teacher sessions or only when the child is in school. If the child resists using them, it may be an indication that they do not fit or function properly, and this possibility should be thoroughly investigated. Having assured yourself in this way, then if constant use is a part of the treatment plan, this should be the goal at home as well as elsewhere.

Essential with either vision or hearing loss is the necessity of devising ways of assisting the flow of information. Further suggestions for doing this will be found in a number of books listed at the end of this chapter. You will devise many of your own ways of adding clues to your child's world as you watch her go about each day. She will also teach you about her world and will devise her own preferred ways to move along the path toward independence.

SOURCES OF ADDITIONAL INFORMATION

Freeman, R.D., et al. *Can't Your Child Hear? A Guide for Those Who Care About Deaf Children.* Baltimore: University Park Press, 1981.
Resource book on deafness, including evidence, opinions, and experiences. Talks about the need for communication and how to implement it. Answers parents' questions and looks at all ages regarding education, deaf culture, and technical aids. Includes sections on multiple disabilities as well as on how to work with professionals.
Kastein, S., et al. *Raising the Young Blind Child: A Guide for Parents and Educators.* New York: Human Sciences Press, 1980.

Suggestions for the care of the blind child up to five years of age. Includes sections on language, motor development, sensory development, and independence training.

17
Children with Severe Disabilities

Severe disability is ordinarily due to marked limitation of functioning in one or more systems of the body. Your child may have limited muscle control that hampers his mobility, his speech, or his ability to feed himself or care for his toileting needs. If either or both vision and hearing are seriously impaired, this may severely limit his ability to function independently. Some degree of mental retardation and seizure activity often accompany severe physical disability or may even represent the major aspect of the disability.

You will need to tailor your expectations for independent functioning to your child's unique set of abilities. This is *not* to say that children who are severely disabled should have no expectations put on them or no attention paid to teaching them. You will note that most of the suggestions and expectations set forth in this book are presented in a gradated form, from simple to more complicated levels. This has been done so that it can serve as a guide for all handicapped persons, with the understanding that those more severely disabled may be

169

limited in the level to which they can progress. Ordinarily, however, those limits are learned only by trial and error, and we are often surprised by what children can do.

Of importance to the child with a severe disability are the obvious personal-care needs, some of which may be intensified because of decreased mobility. The immobile child will need more time for assistance with dressing, eating, bathing, and moving about. The child affected by multiple sensory impairments will need additional time and effort for building communication. If reasoning ability severely limits your child's capacity to interpret and make judgments about his surroundings, this will mean that more time will need to be spent in setting up and supervising an environment that is safe and stimulating.

This level of care is physically and emotionally demanding of parents. In addition, you may at first be disappointed that this is not what you expected in a child. The total effect can be overwhelming at times. For this and other reasons, it is critical that parents of children with severe disability seek assistance in caring for them. This assistance should take several forms. You should take advantage of every source of consultation available (members of your treatment team such as the occupational and physical therapists, other disability specialists, child training organizations, other parents) to learn about basic care and handling techniques, adaptive equipment and services available. As you develop a routine of care and activity you should see that others in the family and eventually child care persons outside the family learn to handle and deal with your child. As you are able to leave the care of your child to others for gradually longer periods of time, this has the obvious advantage of giving you some time for yourself and the less obvious (but equally important) advantage of helping your child to become more flexible. It introduces him to the idea of dealing with different kinds of people.

Additional care is *very* important for you as parents because of the added physical and emotional drain that occurs when caring for a child with a severe disability. It will allow you to have other activities that will help you to gain perspective and enlarge yourself as a person, which will make the time spent with your child more positive. Children with limited skills who have not been cared for by others from early stages can present major problems when changes in routine must occur (such as parents' need to be away or illness of parent or other sibling). It is easy to get trapped into doing it all yourself rather than seeking and teaching competent care workers, and you should not feel that you need to do it all. Should you find yourself with strong feelings of resentment or anger over your situation, seek assistance in dealing with these feelings. Do not try to carry the weight of the world on your shoulders alone.

Sharing responsibility for care is important in that it will allow you to spend time with your mate and your other children. Siblings can grow to resent the disabled child because of the demands on the parents, and you should let them know that such feelings are not bad but are understandable and acceptable. "Feeding Johnny takes a long time, doesn't it, Jerry? Well, I'm almost through, and we'll look at that book you wanted to show me."

If your child is limited in his ability to explore his environment, it will be important that opportunities be provided for stimulation. If he is unable to move voluntarily, he should be placed in different positions during the day so that he can see his world from different angles; in this way he can watch you at your work,

his siblings at play, or look at the TV or out the window.
There are many devices that are helpful to your child. A
variety of wheelchairs, seats, and strollers are available, and
there are many pieces of equipment that are easily made
in the home. Consult your physical and occupational
therapists about choosing appropriate equipment before
you go to a commercial provider. Have the therapists
monitor the fitting of commercial or homemade equipment.

Children should have some structure to their day so
that there is time for play and time for learning. Again,
the larger the variety of settings that are introduced, the
more flexibility will be established. Children often love
the repetition of songs and stories, and records and commercial or home-taped materials are useful learning tools.

The child with mental retardation who also has an
impairment in vision or hearing will often have less
effective use of those senses because his limited reasoning ability has not allowed him to put together the
meaning of what he sees or hears. The child with a
severe seizure disorder might take more time to learn a
task because the disturbance by the seizure may affect
his ability to attend and remember and thus to make
sense of what he sees and hears.

While the child with a severe disability may not be
able to achieve all the levels of independent functioning
outlined for other children, there will be areas in which
his unique capacities can be developed and used. Mothers of all children soon learn what certain looks or body
movements mean, and this is true even with children
whose means of active communication are limited. These
looks and movements are reinforced and given meaning
when we respond to them, and thus will be used again.

By giving your child some way in which to convey his feelings, wants, and needs, his ability to communicate is extended. There are ingenious switches available today that can be activated with minimal pressure to turn on all sorts of things from moving toys to tape recorders to call buttons. For those who are mentally competent but physically limited, wheelchairs can be operated by switches, which may need only slight pressure from the head or hand. Earl was a normally developing boy who was seriously injured in an accident. He is confined to a wheelchair and dependent for all care. He has some use of one arm and hand. He has no speech but can see and hear. He was gradually taught a pointing response whereby he makes choices by pointing to pictures of activities, such as eating, drinking, or particular toys. He was also taught to operate switches for toys that he enjoys. It is a delight to see him in control of a toy airplane that would go fast or slow, up or down, or loop-de-loop with only a slight pressure from his hand. It was clear that the control was as important to Earl as was looking at the plane.

So far we have talked about the severely disabled child in the home. In many communities there exist facilities for training and stimulation outside the home. Most school districts have classrooms for children who are severely disabled or multihandicapped, and as a parent, you should take advantage of whatever appropriate facilities are available. It's a little scary to see your physically dependent child transported to another place and cared for by others there, but the risks are small and the rewards are great. First, it provides some needed time for your personal respite and for attention to other family members. Second, it provides opportunities for your child to learn to be handled by others, to trust them, and to be comfortable in other settings. Third, it provides the opportunity for specialized stimulation and training to occur. If your child is exposed to others, first as caretakers, then in special classrooms, he is more likely as a teenager and young adult to be able to enjoy experiences with peer groups outside the home. These are frequently available as social, recreational, or work activity programs that may be offered by a variety of public or private organizations.

Sometimes the care of a child with a severe disability is simply too difficult for a family. There may be family illness, there may be inadequate assistance because of limited finances or because help is simply not available, or other good reasons why it may be difficult to maintain the child in the home. In such cases, parents can seek residential care on a short-term or long-term basis. Some facilities offer short-term (two weeks to a month) residence on a respite care basis. Other facilities specialize in the care and training of those with severe physical and mental limitations on a long-term basis. Residential placement may have some advantage for enhancing the quality of life of your child. He will be able to enjoy peer interaction that will not have been available at home. We all need a chance to identify with others, to compete on a basis so that we can sometimes win, and to be in a situation where we are not always the "sore thumb." The facilities and services available in residential settings also may offer a greater span of specialized services than could be available in individual settings. If you think such placement may represent the best overall option for your child and your family, then seek information about it, including details about any financial assistance that might be available. There are often waiting lists for such centers. Your state mental health division or other social service agencies may assist you in planning for such a placement. You can assist your residentially placed child by becoming familiar with his program and the organization administering it, by regular visits, and by monitoring his health and progress. You should not see this as giving up on your child if you have carefully considered all available options and conclude that residential placement is best for him.

SOURCES OF ADDITIONAL INFORMATION

Burkhart, L.J. *More Homemade Battery Devices for Severely Handicapped Children with Suggested Activities*, 1982. Write: Linda J. Burkhart, RD 1, Box 124, Millville, Pa 17846.
Ingenious devices to help severely disabled children interact with their environment.

Finnie, N.R. *Handling the Young Cerebral Palsied Child at Home*. New York: E.P. Dutton, 1975.
A guide to teaching adaptive behavior skills to very young children with serious motor limitations. Includes chapters on sleeping, toilet training, dressing, and feeding as well as other areas.

Hale, G., ed. *The Source Book for the Disabled: An Illustrated Guide to Easier More Independent Liv-*

ing for Physically Disabled People, Their Families and Friends. New York: Bantam, 1981.

A comprehensive how-to book with sections on daily living skills, leisure and recreation, sexuality, and other relevant topics. Includes an extended list of resource organizations and publications.

Roberts, S., and N. Sydow. *Consumer's Guide to Attendant Care.* Access to Independence, Inc.: Madison, Wisconsin, 1984.

A step-by-step guide for assessing the need for an attendant, advertising for and hiring an attendant, training and utilizing the services of an attendant.

18

The Single Parent

The circumstances that lead to raising a child alone are several. You may be separated, divorced, or never married. You may be the biological or the adoptive parent. Parenthood may be a goal that you have achieved after careful deliberation, or it may have been unanticipated. While many of the issues of raising a family by yourself are the same as raising a family with another person, you might well have a different perspective if the situation is one that you have chosen rather than one that was thrust upon you.

Single parenthood is frequently not a matter of choice. The spouse may have died, a divorce may have not been anticipated or desired, or the child may have been the result of a pregnancy that had no real involvement of the biological partner following conception. A parent may sometimes desert because of disappointment at having a disabled child or because of inability to deal with an anticipated emotional and financial strain in rearing the child. Natalie and Don's child was normal at birth but was left with severe disabilities following an episode of seizures as an infant. They were a young couple who had had the usual expectations for what their family would be like in ten years, and when these expectations were shattered, Don simply couldn't handle it, left, and obtained a divorce. Natalie had not been employed prior to the marriage. She had a lot of family support and guts, and she pursued business training and became employed. She received support from family and friends and in time worked out a realistic balance between care for her child and a life of her own.

A large proportion of the problems for the single parent revolve around the time needed to fulfill the considerable duties involved in parenting. In a two-parent family those obligations are usually divided to some extent, while the single parent has to meet all the needs of the family. It is demanding and difficult to be both the provider and caregiver without assistance or relief. Where the two-parent family can share decision making about problems of child rearing (or in the case of disability, about treatment), the single parent has to make most of the decisions without a ready source of consultation, support, or assistance. The result may be a drain on the physical and emotional well-being of the single parent.

From the start, you should arrange help with baby-sitting and respite care for your child. This is an important step for a two-parent family, and it is doubly important for a single parent. It should be set up early, in the form of help from a trusted friend, relative, or mature sitter. This starts the exposure of the child to handling by other adults, and that is particularly critical when such exposure is not going to be so easily available. For you the parent this provides some relief from the physical and emotional demands of child care and should help give a sense of perspective. Time away can also provide the opportunity for some degree of normal social life and relief from loneliness.

Maintaining an adequate level of employment may also become an issue because the single parent has fewer options in responding to emergency situations, such as illness, that may arise with children during the working day. This may place limits on the type, stability, and wage level of the employment available to her or him. There may be more than one child in the home, and this adds to the problem, particularly when the children are small. The best single approach to this difficult problem is to broaden your support network as much as possible. This may include family, the other parent, friends, neighbors, day care arrangements (some are now available for sick children), multiple babysitters, respite care providers, disability-related support organizations, and single parent organizations. Seek them out, pay your dues (literal and figurative) by becoming part and supporting *them* (organizations and friendships), and turn to them as occasional sources of help in ordinary times as well as in emergencies.

Support groups can provide emotional support as well as assistance with details of caring for your child. They will often have meetings at which child care is provided so that both you and your child can benefit from social contact. Single parent organizations can be particularly supportive in providing social and recreational opportunities. It will be useful to create patterns of socializing both with and without your disabled child. You each need social contact, and separate activities will keep you in touch with adults as well as provide expanded social experiences for your child.

Other hazards that can be part of single parenthood are intense loneliness (particularly for adult company), feelings of rejection, bitterness at the situation, and boredom with a demanding routine. Overeating and its consequences are a common pitfall for the beleagured single parent. It is important that your support network include at least one person who is a trusted confidant or consultant. There are times when you may want to express loneliness, fear, frustration, and anger. There are other times when you may simply want to bat around an idea or decision with another adult. You may be lucky enough to have several persons with whom you can do this or to whom you can go for different purposes. They might include family, friends, or religious counselors. They should be able to listen without themselves panicking, without expecting to solve every problem, and without trying to control you. Should you find yourself without such support, you may want to seek the help of a professional social worker, psychologist, or counselor. This may be on a regular or occasional basis. It is commonly done by people in stressful situations or who find themselves confronting difficult decisions. It does not mean that your emotional health is anything less than normal for the situation. It may mean that you are a wise person. The stakes for you and your children are considerable.

A particular pitfall in single parenthood is that of making the child the confidant for adult matters. It is easy but unwise to unload difficulties on your child simply because she is easily available. This particularly pertains to sharing problems over which the child has no control. A child may become fearful or feel guilty when she knows that the rent is overdue or that Mom is having trouble at work, even though she is powerless to help with the solution. This is not to say that your child should be unrealistically sheltered and spoiled, but that a good deal of judgment should be used in deciding what problems should be shared and how they should be presented. This also underscores the necessity of having some other adult or a counselor with whom you can share your worries and frustrations. You and your child have the opportunity for a closer, and possible richer, relationship just between the two of you. The trick is to prevent it from becoming a relationship that is over-dependent or that restricts either of you in your social growth.

A trap absolutely to be avoided is that of sharing a bed with your child, and the earlier this separation is made, the better. This situation can be a particularly difficult one for the single parent (and the child) in that they may strongly feel the need for warmth and closeness. Children who have discomfort from disability or illness may need your presence and comforting to go to sleep, but this should be done without your presence in the bed. Parents can become caught in this pattern of lying down with the child, and it is easier to break it earlier than later. Your child will become a more flexible person, and you will have less difficulty in emergency situations (if you or your child are ill or hospitalized). Your own privacy should be respected, and the stage for this should be set early rather than later, in possibly embarrassing circumstances.

There are a number of problems that may arise for the *children* of single parents. There can be a risk of emotional neglect, simply because of the amount of time that is needed to provide for the basic requirements of the family. The pressures make those quiet, intimate times hard to come by and make the patience needed for teaching a scarce commodity. This situation also increases the possibility of child abuse. I'm-at-the-end-of-my-rope feelings often occur when you do not have the safety valve of another adult to listen or to ease matters by taking over a difficult situation. Again, the availability of a support network or confidant is important. *It is especially important that you seek help if you begin to feel that you cannot control negative feelings toward your child.*

School-aged children are susceptible to school phobia (abnormal aversion toward school), which can have its roots in a fear of loss of the remaining parent, with consequent anxiety about being away from him or her. Children being raised by a single parent sometimes become the focus of that parent's attention, become spoiled, and need and demand constant attention. A great deal of time spent with the parent may also deprive them of the interaction with peers by which they can learn the social skills needed for adolescent and adult living. The adolescent child of a single parent (and the parent) may find being separated more difficult at a time when striving for independence is a natural drive. The adolescent may have conflict about rebelling against her only source of support, and the parent in turn may experience heightened feelings of rejection at this time. Finally there is the obvious lack of the sex role model usually provided by the other parent. In the single parent situation, it is typically the mother who has the responsibility of the child rearing, while the male role model is absent or inadequately represented. This absence may hamper the child's ability to form an accurate perception of that sex role. The reverse may of course be true if the single parent is male.

It is a good idea to avoid moving your place of residence, if possible. It is difficult for children (as well as adults) to make friends in new neighborhoods, and this may be doubly difficult if your child has a disability that makes her appear different from other children. Frequent moves disrupt schooling and make it particularly difficult if your child needs special services. School stability will make your child's life easier.

If you are a single parent you should be clear about your legal rights as they pertain to your children. If there is a divorce where there are custodial issues, be sure you are clear about them. The same is true for issues of adoption. As children of a single parent, your children would also profit by your foresightedness in making contingency plans for matters such as illness or death. Because there is often not another legal parent involved, such things as a will and clear insurance arrangements become increasingly important.

Further suggestions for the single parent can be found in the references at the end of this chapter. The problems of the single parent of the child with a disability are not all that different from those of any single parent, just more intensified. Seeking babysitting help early, maintaining social contacts, finding a confidant, and avoiding isolating traps are of the utmost importance to single parent families.

SOURCES OF ADDITIONAL INFORMATION

S.D.K. "I feel like I'm dealing with these problems all by myself: Demands on single parents." *The Exceptional Parent,* Vol. 12, pp. 43–49.

  Account of one single parent family, the difficulties they encountered in rearing a disabled child, and some helpful actions they took.

Greywolf, E.S. *The Single Mother's Handbook.* New York: Morrow, 1984.

  This book is about single motherhood in general. It looks at meeting the new situation and finding ways of dealing with the problems of stress, time, money, and employment.

19

For the Parent

Rearing a child is not an easy task. It is much more art than science. There is plenty of room for you to have your own style, and because all of the answers are not known, there is plenty of opportunity to use your own judgment. This is a mixed blessing. Sometimes it would be nice to have more answers. To do your best in good faith is what is needed, and to be tolerant of yourself as you muddle through some difficult situations. Many others have done it before you. This is especially true for the first child, but even experienced parents will recognize that they have muddled through, even with second and third children, each of whom will present his own set of problems. So—look for guidance rather than answers, from others with experience, from books, from professionals, and from your own past experiences. Beware of set answers for all occasions. In the end you will need to make your own judgments, and it matters most that they are made in the best interest of the child. It is a happy fact that children (and people), with or without disability, tend to be durable and resilient.

Having a child with a disability may increase your responsibilities in several ways: some of the problems can be more complex and may require information or advice from professionals, and often the total burden of care amounts to more than it would with a nondisabled child. At times this matter of extra time and patience can become a touchy one, as we heard from one parent who said, "Please don't tell me *again* that the only way my child [cerebral palsied] will learn to dress himself is if I take the time to give him the practice! I know that, and I do it most of the time, but it can be very frustrating!" Frustration with time pressures and guilt about frustration can be a cycle that can build up for parents and may need to be resolved by some counseling for conflict resolution and/or schedule adjustment to deal with the time element. Also, you are entitled now and again to blow off steam at so-called experts who get a bit preachy.

These are some of the reasons that make it desirable to spread out the care of your disabled child, accepting and using the help of others. This should start within the family, so that one person does not become the sole caretaker for the child. Relatives and friends will often be glad to help in specific ways, such as providing care for an hour, a day, or a weekend. In some communities there are organized systems for providing respite care or attendant services through public or private agencies. They are there because others recognize the need for parents and siblings to have time for activities that may not be appropriate for the disabled child. Far from feeling guilty, you should see such respite or "vacations" as a means of maintaining the family as a healthy, wholesome, and interesting group context in which the disabled child can grow. Each of the members of the family (including the disabled person) is entitled to a life of his own as well as a life within the family.

There is no question that having a member with a

severe disability will place some burden on all of the family because of the need to provide care, modify some activities, and quite possibly use funds for treatment rather than for other family purposes. There is, however, no justification for making a martyr of the family or any of its members. When a person, such as the mother, dedicates the entirety of her life to the child, the end result is ordinarily not good for the child, for the rest of the family, or for the martyred person. There is too much opportunity for narrowing the focus of activities. The caregiver finds it difficult to avoid being overcontrolling or guilt-ridden. Sam's mother responded with "What kind of a mother will they think I am?" every time it was suggested that Sam's (sometimes sloppy) grooming and self-care was good enough for going to school and that he would improve with practice. As a result she is still shaving him every day at age twenty-three, although he could—and should—be doing it himself.

Feelings of guilt or resentment may frequently be present, whether or not they are stated, in other members of the family. This can be prevented by spreading the burden of care around, accepting help from many sources, and also by talking about feelings within the family. It is important to make it possible for persons to say when they feel overburdened or unfairly used. It is especially important that family members find someone to turn to if they begin to direct their negative feelings toward the child.

It is apparent that maintaining a marriage or any ongoing, stable, male-female relationship has become difficult in our society. Responsibility for children adds stress to that, and responsibility for a disabled child increases the stress. If there are two of you, it is important that it be a partnership: burdens should be shared and responsibilities shifted from time to time; you should attempt to pick up for your spouse when things become overwhelming; and you should freely and regularly discuss the functioning of the family. There is no situation in which it is justified to hold one parent responsible for the disability and all its attendant care. Where there is significant conflict that continues over time, as may occur in the family that has added stress, you would be well advised to obtain professional counseling from a person such as a psychologist, social worker, or minister trained in dealing with problems of stressed families.

As the child grows up one of the more difficult matters to handle is that of the attitudes that may be held toward him by others, both within and outside the family. Persons with disability may have attributes that quite markedly differ from those that are generally found: they may look different, they may walk awkwardly, or their speech may be difficult to understand. There is a tendency within the family to ignore these things because you grow accustomed to them and because you know the person's strong and positive qualities, which may not be as obvious as the negative ones. These facts of disability should not be the focus of every discussion with the child, but neither should such discussion be systematically avoided. For them never to be discussed suggests that they are matters for embarrassment or shame and allows both the positive and negative feelings to remain unspoken on the part of the disabled child, his siblings, or you the parents. Each of you, and especially the disabled child, needs to have some familiarity with the fact that he is different in the way that he looks, walks, or talks. This should lead to a balanced view of his qualities, both positive and negative. It should also help him, as well as the rest of the family, work out strategies to handle the occasional negative reactions of strangers, from staring to teasing to outright rejection. Hopefully the qualities of your handicapped child (as well as unusual characterisitics of other family members) can be a matter of open discussion that will lead to a healthy perspective and to a sense of humor to ease some of the difficult moments and make life just a bit more pleasant.

Making life a bit more pleasant could be identified as the theme of this short chapter. You have a tough job, and it will be easier if it is shared. Expect some difficult moments, and congratulate yourself and your child when you survive. After a particularly stressful time, treat yourself to something nice. Try to balance stressful things with pleasant things. Each of you is entitled to a life of his or her own, and to enjoy it!

Appendix

PORTLAND TRACKING SYSTEM
FOR ADULT LIVING

Date_____
Name_____
BD _____ Age _____
Filled out by_____
Agency_____

	Status				Comments/Action
	Acquired	Needs Attention	Uncertain	Not Applicable	
I. PERSONAL SURVIVAL					
A. Body Maintenance					
1. Cleans self					
2. Grooms					
3. Keeps physically fit					
4. Cares for self when sick					
5. Can get professional help when needed					
6. Prepares and serves nutritious food					
7. Orders meals in restaurants					
8. Dresses self and maintains clothing					
9. Maintains safety and personal security					
10. Handles emergencies					
B. Home and Equipment Maintenance					
1. Cleans house					
2. Manages household repairs					
3. Shops for household items					
4. Can locate a place to live					
5. Locks doors and windows					

PORTLAND TRACKING SYSTEM FOR ADULT LIVING

	Status				Comments/Action
Date_____ Name_____ BD_____ Age_____ Filled out by_____ Agency_____	Acquired	Needs Attention	Uncertain	Not Applicable	
6. Maintains adaptive equipment					
C. Money Management					
1. Budgets money					
2. Uses bank					
3. Makes change					
D. Mobility Ability					
1. Copes with architectural barriers					
2. Walks or uses wheelchair					
3. Uses transportation (car/bus)					
4. Finds way around community					
5. Carries items					
E. Time					
1. Tells time					
2. Manages time					
F. Communication					
1. Talks/uses phone					
2. Writes/uses post office					
3. Asks for help when needed					
4. Communicates nonverbally					

PORTLAND TRACKING SYSTEM
FOR ADULT LIVING

Date_____
Name_____
BD_____ Age_____
Filled out by_____
Agency_____

	Acquired	Needs Attention	Uncertain	Not Applicable	Comments/Action
II. SOCIAL					
A. Initiates activities and makes choices					
B. Uses the appropriate behavior for the situation					
C. Has appropriate sexual behavior and knowledge					
D. Has friends					
E. Has appropriate dating behavior					
F. Participates in groups					
G. Manages continued social contacts					
H. Has individual actitivies and personal recreation					
I. Has good relationship with parents					
J. Asserts self when needed					
K. Knows rights and acts responsibly					
III. VOCATIONAL					
A. Has basic educational skills, i.e., reading, writing, arithmetic					
B. Has good work habits					
C. Has marketable work skills					
D. Can apply for a job					

PORTLAND TRACKING SYSTEM
FOR ADULT LIVING

		Acquired	Needs Attention	Uncertain	Not Applicable	Comments/Action
	Status					
Date_____ Name_____ BD_____ Age_____ Filled out by_____ Agency_____						
	E. Has had work experience					
	F. Has been competitively employed					
	G. Has vocational plans					
	H. Has realistic awareness of vocational strengths and weaknesses.					
IV. OTHER						

Index

<pre></pre>

JAMES E. LINDEMANN earned his Ph.D. in Clinical Psychology from Pennsylvania State University in 1954, and is now Professor of Medical Psychology in the Crippled Children's Division of the Oregon Health Sciences University. In addition to helping handicapped children and their families cope with disabilities, Dr. Lindemann specializes in career counseling and the problems of adolescents. The author of *Psychological and Behavioral Aspects of Physical Disability*, he has served on the advisory or governing boards of community organizations involved with cerebral palsy, hemophilia, rehabilitation, child and family services, and suicide prevention. Dr. Lindemann is also a Fellow of the American Psychological Association.

SALLY J. LINDEMANN holds a bachelor's degree from Ohio Wesleyan University and a master of science degree in Clinical Psychology from Pennsylvania State University. Since 1974, she has been a school psychologist with the District and Regional Assessment Center of the Portland School District, where she is involved in evaluating the educational and support needs of those children who are candidates for pre-school and school programs.